The Butterfly and Life Span Nutrition

Principles and practice of life span nutrition based on intuitive insights of the ancients and an understanding of the molecular dynamics of health and disease

How to eat life span foods to lose weight and enjoy greater energy, better health and longer life

Majid Ali, M.D.

Associate Professor of Pathology (Adj)
Columbia University, New York
Director, Department of Pathology, Immunology and Laboratories
Holy Name Hospital, Teaneck, New Jersey
Consulting Physician
Institute of Preventive Medicine, Denville, New Jersey
Fellow, Royal College of Surgeons of England
Diplomate, American Board of Environmental Medicine

Library of Congress Cataloging-in-Publication Data

Ali, Majid
The Butterfly and Life Span Nutrition Majid Ali.--1st ed.

Includes bibliographical references and index
1. Life Span Nutrition
2. Life Span Foods
3. Aging-Oxidant Foods
4. Nature of Obesity and Weight Loss
5. The Catabolic Maladaptation
6. Up-regulation of Fat-burning Enzymes

TXU 535-766   1992   ISBN 1-879131-01-3
10 9 8 7 6 5 4 3 2 1

Published in the USA by

Institute of Preventive Medicine
95 East Main Street, Denville, N.J 07843
(201) 586-4111

Dedicated to those who asked me
to be their physician, and so honored me.

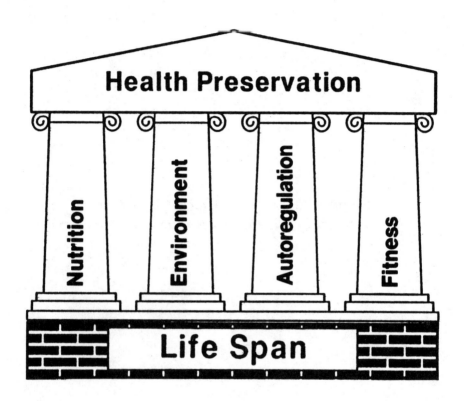

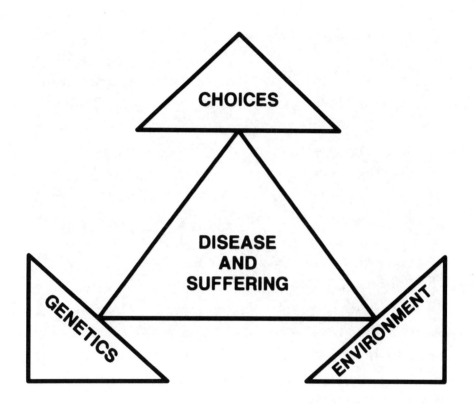

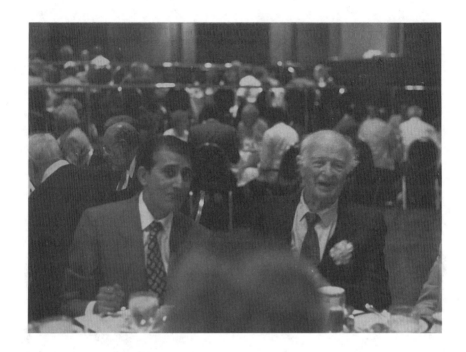

The author with Linus Pauling at the spring 1992 conference of
the American College for Advancement in Medicine in Dallas,
where he presented Pauling the annual Achievement Award of
the College. Pauling is the only American to receive two
unshared Nobel prizes.

Acknowledgments

I am grateful to my patients who considered the principles of life span nutrition outlined in this book and validated them by their true-to-life experiences; to my colleagues in nutritional medicine and environmental medicine, too numerous to name here, who listened and critiqued my concepts of the essential chemistry of life and my notions of life span and aging-oxidant foods as I presented them at the conferences of the American Academy of Environmental Medicine, American Academy of Otolaryngic Allergy and the American College for Advancement in Medicine; to Ronald Russo and his staff at the library of Holy Name Hospital, Teaneck, New Jersey, for their unfailing support; to Jerrold Finnie, M.D., Dolores Finnie, R.N., Maria Sumberac and Lois Roselli for their editorial work; to my publisher at the Institute of Preventive Medicine, Denville, New Jersey; and to my wife, Talat, who has the persuasion of a scientist and the patience of a saint.

Contents

Preface

One of my patients suffered from incapacitating chronic fatigue, multiple allergies and chemical sensitivity. She rapidly gained about 30 pounds after she developed this ailment. I asked her once how she thought this may have happened. She replied,

> *"Dr. Ali, I know my whole metabolism has shut down."*

Did her metabolism really shut down? How could such a thing have happened? These questions have long since stayed with me. Many of my other patients with indolent immune and degenerative disorders gained weight rapidly after becoming ill. They also spoke of a "sluggish" or "suppressed" metabolism and "poisoned" or "toxic" cells. Do their cells really become poisoned? Or toxic? Of course, in classical drug medicine we are taught to vigorously dismiss such "patient fantasies." Among physicians, such notions are regarded as fodder for the feebleminded. Nevertheless, I simply could not dismiss these questions and searched for ways to restore my patients' deranged molecular pathways and ease their suffering.

Could this be a delusional plausibility? Tremors of troubled minds? Search for false hopes?

Or are there some deep intuitive insights buried in such "simplistic" ideas? Some profound visceral understanding of human metabolic and energy pathways? Are they hallucinating or are they truly sensing some down-regulation or even arrest of their enzyme systems?

Most people with immune disorders and chronic fatigue lose weight when they are successfully managed with nutrient therapies, allergy treatment and self-regulation. How does this take place?

"Ulooo the puthee kuuht khaiey."

Silly girl, why doesn't she eat less, I heard a Pakistani say once as she watched a very obese woman talk about the perils of obesity on a talk show. Is it really that simple? All an obese person has to do to become thin is to eat less? Who is right, my patient with chronic fatigue who thinks her whole metabolism has shut down, or this Pakistani woman? I know of many dieting "experts" and physicians who will agree with the woman from Pakistan. I must admit this is how I myself often thought during my early heady days in surgery. A surgical mind sees things differently. Fat is made up of calories. Calories come from food. It should follow that an obese person should lose unwanted pounds of fat by simply eating less. End of discussion.

Two Observations of the Ancients

The ancients made two basic observations about human

metabolism.

First,

the ancients knew that metabolism can be slowed down by fasting (the ancient equivalent of modern dieting). They recognized and expounded the need for this during periods of reflection, meditation, prayer and silence.

Second,

the ancients knew that metabolism can be accelerated by eating and with physical exercise. Food fuels the furnace of human metabolism; exercise stokes its fire.

Both truths are self-evident. All we need to do is to test them. The ancients, of course, could not foresee the chemical avalanches we would unleash upon our metabolism. As intuitive as they were, they could not have foreseen the case of metabolism shut down by synthetic aging-oxidant molecules.

Our nutrition and diet experts, it seems to me, do not have much respect either for the intuitive wisdom of the ancients or for the science of molecular structure and function. I suspect this is so because such elements do not support the profitability goals of the merchants of our dieting industry and their "experts." They are determined to put all of us on their packaged frozen (and toxic) foods.

I have been a student of medicine for about 35 years. As a hospital pathologist during the last 25 years, I have personally examined close to 90,000 biopsies and surgical specimens. The microscope helps us define and classify diseases clearly. We have learned to treat acute diseases as defined by the microscope with great skill, precision and safety. During the early years of my pathology work, it became clear to me that the microscope has serious limitations when it comes to chronic diseases. The microscope can only help us to look at the tail end of disease, when the tissue damage has already been done. The microscope does not allow us to look at the front end of disease, before the tissues have been damaged. This is the principal lesson taught to me by my microscope.

What do we do if we do not wish to limit our work to looking at the tail ends of diseases? What do we do if we seek to look at the front ends of diseases? The answer for me has been molecular medicine. I quote below a brief passage from my book *The Cortical Monkey and Healing.*

> *"I use the term molecular medicine to refer to a practice of medicine based on molecular events which occur before cells and tissues are injured by the disease. Molecular medicine is not based upon what we observe in cells with a microscope after the cells have been damaged. In molecular medicine, treatment protocols are formulated based upon the knowledge of the structure and function of molecules and the molecular requirements of the patient; the science of outcome studies substantiates the validity of these protocols."*

In my clinical work in molecular medicine, I care for my patients with integrated treatment protocols of nutritional medicine, environmental medicine, medicine of self-regulation and medicine of fitness. This work has given me some new insights into the molecular and energy bases of health and disease. This work has also given me a compelling sense of holistic molecular relatedness in human biology. Two questions have preoccupied me during these years:

What poisons and paralyzes energy enzymes? How can poisoned enzymes be brought back to life?

In this book, and in its companion volume *The Canary and Chronic Fatigue*, several observations are made which throw light on these two questions. I begin here with a brief outline of the essentials of chemistry and biology of life in nature.

Molecular Duality of Oxygen

What is the essential chemistry of life in man? What are the basic designs and mechanisms in human biology? What are the fundamentals of health, aging, disease and death? These are the central issues for those interested in the healing arts. There is a paradox here. Much is known to our colleagues in chemistry and physics about these subjects. However, little, if any, of it is used in the prevailing mode of drug medicine in the United States.

Oxygen brings forth life. Oxygen sustains life. Oxygen terminates life. Oxygen builds molecules. Oxygen lacerates, mutilates and destroys molecules.

Oxygen is a molecular Dr. Jekyll and Mr. Hyde. The beneficial effects of oxygen are generally well known. Yet, the toxic effects of oxygen are rarely appreciated.

Spontaneity of oxidation, it seems to me, is the essential nature of the chemistry of life, health, aging and disease.

A petal of a flower withers away in a few days. This occurs because the molecules in the petal are oxidized. Chopped lettuce turns brown within hours. This is due to oxidation of the lettuce leaves. An apple falls off a tree and bruises its skin in one area. The next day that area spoils. This is also a result of oxidation. Oxidation in nature is a spontaneous process. It needs no outside programming. In chemical language, oxidation is loss of electrons (the tiniest packets of energy) by molecules in all matter. It is the nature of high-energy molecules to lose electrons (get oxidized) and settle down to a lower level of energy.

All living organisms have powerful oxidant molecules that can cause immediate self-combustion of the organism, unless of course their destructive capacity is held in check by other molecules. I call these oxidant molecules "aging-oxidant molecules."

A piece of iron is thrown into a stream of water. Some days later, it turns brown. Rusting of iron is also a form of oxidation. Rust, in chemistry jargon, is known as iron oxide. Thus, oxidation is as much a part of what we consider the inanimate world as it is of the animal and plant kingdoms.

Spontaneity of oxidation is nature's grand design for not allowing any form of life to live forever. What would happen if any single form of life were immune to the law of death in nature? Our planet Earth would be packed with that form of life (and its offspring) and there would be no room left for any other life form. There would be no space for a new flower to bloom or a new baby to be born.

A mosquito dies after 18 days. The tissues of a mouse disintegrate after two years. A monkey lives for 18 years. The life expectancy of man is estimated to be about 110 years. Why do different species have different life spans? A mosquito can live for 18 days because that is how long his tissues can resist oxidation. The tissues and molecules of a mosquito resist progressive oxidation by producing another family of molecules that counteract the aging-oxidant molecules. I call these molecules "life span molecules."

The earmark of life in our time is accelerated oxidative molecular stress on human biology.

Environmental pollutants are oxidant molecules. Pesticides, herbicides and fungicides are "designer" killer molecules. They are powerful oxidant molecules. Pervasive use of antibiotics is increasing oxidant stress on human tissues -- directly, because antibiotics are designed to kill life, and indirectly, because antibiotics seriously damage the ecology of the gut. Highly processed foods increase oxidant stress on tissues. Lack of physical fitness causes musculoskeletal restrictions, persistent muscle spasms, and increased oxidant stress on tissues. Finally, adrenaline and related stress molecules are powerful oxidant molecules.

Excessive oxidant stress causes molecular burnout. Aging occurs at an accelerated rate. Tissues hurt and despair. The cells agonize and die. Diseases begin to take shape. Death looms large. *This is the single most important insight my patients have given me.*

Degenerative diseases and chronic immune disorders, at energy and molecular levels, are consequences of accelerated oxidative molecular injury. The words of my patient who considered her metabolism shut down by events which caused chronic fatigue reflect her enormous intuitive insight. She *knew* what had happened to her metabolism, in a deep visceral way. I have often wondered how easy it would be for us physicians to make correct diagnoses for our patients if only we would *listen* to them. This patient made me see more clearly than ever the absolute need to break through the barriers imposed upon me by my microscope. I realized I must learn to look at "diseases" differently if I were going to have the opportunity to unravel the mystery of shut-down metabolism.

Obesity is a state of down-regulated enzymes. The central question for me has been this: How does one bring back to life the poisoned and paralyzed enzymes, or, in the words of another one of my patients, how does one "open the metabolism?"

Obesity is not a problem of the mind. It is a matter of poisoned enzymes, and of clogged molecular wheels of metabolism. The enzymes of an obese person do not get poisoned because his mother did not hug him enough. His enzymes were poisoned by toxic foods. His molecular wheels didn't get clogged because his father neglected to say "I love you" enough times. Rather, they were clogged by the toxins in the water he drank and the air he breathed. His lipase enzymes didn't become sluggish because he suppressed his anger as a child. Every additional pound of fat that he accumulated further suppressed his enzymes in a direct linear relationship. This is now well established.

The solution to obesity is to heed the intuitive wisdom of the ancients and to know the structure and function of nutrient molecules and synthetic toxins that modern science gives us. Some segments of this book may seem tedious to those uninitiated in the basics of modern science. However, I am confident that once the reader grasps the basic equation of aging-oxidant and life span molecules of life as I describe here, it will be easy for him to sift true useful nutritional information from the huge body of worthless verbiage which passes for nutrition "science."

Two Nutrition Sciences

Nutrition knowledge in the United States comes in two

broad categories:

Nutrition knowledge of the practitioners of nutritional medicine who seek to reverse chronic diseases and prevent illness with nutritional therapies; and

Nutrition knowledge of the practitioners of drug medicine who, by their own admission, do not practice nutritional medicine and yet consider the practice of nutritional medicine quackery.

The latter group usually conducts "research" by feeding mice or medical students this or that nutrient for four or six weeks and thinks its conclusions have absolute validity for the whole life span of all human beings. Since such studies mostly generate contradictory data, the medical profession at large is convinced nutrients have no real value in the treatment of disease except what they narrowly define as "deficiency" diseases.

The nutrition "science" of the practitioners of drug medicine is of no interest to the serious student of biology. The practitioners of drug medicine are focused on disease. Their "nutrition science" is of no value to either overweight people or those in the throes of chronic illness.

The subjects of health, vigor and optimal weight for the whole human life span cannot be separated from the second important intuitive wisdom of the ancients: the need for physical activity to up-regulate the metabolism. In the companion volume, *The Ghoraa and Limbic Exercise,* I draw heavily from the intuitive wisdom of the ancients as well as the true science of the biologist. Again, I have unceremoniously dismissed the "science" of our exercise experts. I have tried to follow the steps of the African message carrier and the Aztec runner. They *knew* something about the exhilaration of running and something about the sacredness of the earth they ran over. They were not into perspiring or hyperventilating. Neither did they carry silly notions of lowering their blood cholesterol levels by running. When they ran, they simply ran. I have also tried to follow the insight of the biologist. He has no hidden agenda. He simply observes things and reports them. The biologist is not into running at 70% of the maximum aerobic capacity and other frivolous notions like that with which the exercise experts are infatuated.

I do not offer any great discoveries of secret exotic potions that "melt the fat away," but rather some basic observations about human metabolism, nutrition, health and disease. I have focused on some essential aspects of the chemistry of aging, fat and sugar metabolism, and the factors that cause down-regulation of enzymes and lead to obesity. Most of all, I have concentrated on ways of using exercise and foods to up-regulate enzyme systems that normally maintain optimal weight. I hope my observations about the nature of obesity and my suggestions for up-regulation of enzymes systems will be of some help to the reader.

In the chapter Life Span Nutrition, I give a detailed

breakdown of foods that support the life span molecules for health, vigor and vitality for the life span of the individual. In that chapter, I also include detailed lists of foods that favor the aging-oxidant molecules. I have attempted to give a blend of the intuitive wisdom and the empirical observations of the ancients and modern science in matters of health, disease and death.

I am not a martyr. I don't like my patients to be martyrs. It is not my purpose to give the reader a dieting plan for achieving and maintaining an optimal weight for the entire life span. Rather, it is my hope that this book will help him or her to develop a philosophy of nutrition and fitness. From extensive clinical work, I *know* that it is possible for all of us to slowly bring about the change that makes doing what we *like* to do the same as what we *need* to do for a healthy long life.

Majid Ali, M.D.
Denville, New Jersey
September 1, 1992.

Chapter 1

The Cortical Monkey, Autoregulation and Molecular Medicine

The Cortical Monkey, Autoregulation
and Molecular Medicine

The terms cortical monkey, autoregulation and molecular medicine appear throughout this book. Following are some excerpts from my previous book, *The Cortical Monkey and Healing,* that will serve as a reference for these terms.

The Cortical Monkey

There is a particular species of monkey native to Karnal, my birthplace. During my childhood, these monkeys lived in our town by the hundreds. They were a nuisance for the grown-ups, but for us children they were a lot of fun. I remember my father telling me how these monkeys had a peculiar habit. They did not let their wounds heal. If one of them ever lacerated his skin, he would pick at his wound continuously. He would peal off whatever little scab did form. These wounds festered for long periods of time.

Putting Something
Between the Monkey And His Wound

It has occurred to me that the first man to invent a

bandage probably got his idea from watching a monkey (or some other animal) constantly pick at his wound. It might have occurred to him that the way to let the wound heal would be to put something between the monkey and his wound. When he got hurt himself, the lesson learned from the monkey might have taken a practical turn. A bunch of leaves, perhaps of some herbal plant, might have served this purpose. This, or something similar, is likely to have been the forerunner of of our modern Band-Aid.

There is something relevant in the story of Karnal monkeys to our ideas of self-regulation and healing. Time and again, I see patients who understand how their *cortical condition* throws roadblocks in the way of *limbic healing*. In our autoregulation laboratory, I demonstrate to them their biologic profiles composed of a host of electro-magnetic or molecular events. I show them how their whole biology is sustained in an even state when they go *limbic*, and how it is thrown into turbulence when they go *cortical*. I explain to them the impact on their internal organs of *talking for control* and *listening for healing*. At intellectual and analytical levels, they seem to understand these phenomena. Yet left to their own devices, they slide back into the calculating and competitive *cortical state*. They are unable to keep their analytical mind ("the cortical monkey") out of the way of the healing *limbic state* .

Indeed, patient and persistent work is required to break long-established cortical habits and put the cortical monkey to sleep.

Thinking is an intellectual function;
healing is not.

In autoregulation, I do not ask my patients to think positively. In autoregulation, I strive to teach them *how not* to think. Thinking about how not to think is a classical catch 22. The harder we try not to think, the deeper we slide into thinking. This is where the concept of energy in autoregulation comes into play.

The theoretical concepts of the value of positive thinking are well understood by most people. The obvious benefits of positive thinking notwithstanding, such thoughts by themselves, in my experience, are rarely sufficient to allow most people to reverse chronic disorders and regain health. Indeed, patients debilitated by chronic diseases and exhausted by unrelenting suffering often find the advice of positive thinking as salt on their wounds. I do not make a practice of this.

The concept of physical healing energy in autoregulation is often misunderstood in a society that is oriented to chemical resolution of all health problems. Many of my patients equate it to some variant of Eastern philosophy or mysticism when I introduce them to the principles and practice of autoregulation. Fortunately, most people are able to perceive this healing energy in some fashion during the very first training session in my autoregulation laboratory. This strips from the concept of healing energy all the layers of disbelief, distrust and apprehension. From then on, it is simply a matter of increasing the intensity of such energy and enhancing its clinical benefits.

*Injured molecules and cells heal with energy.
Autoregulation is about this energy.*

The critical issue is how to become aware of this energy, how to increase its intensity and, finally, how to use it to regulate one's biology and allow the injured molecules and cells to heal. In the initial stages, it is necessary to understand clearly *what autoregulation is and what it is not.*

* *Autoregulation is healing by listening to tissues and perceiving their energy.*

* *Autoregulation is not healing by talking to tissues and thinking positively.*

The principles of self-regulation are valid for all patients and all diseases. The applications of these principles, however, require careful evaluation of each individual patient to assess the nature and extent of his disease (weight and duration of the specific burdens on his biology). Different diseases cause different levels of suffering and require different degrees of effort with different time frames.

In my early clinical work with environmental medicine,

I saw patients who responded poorly or not at all to the standard drug therapies. Many of them were actually made worse by drugs. Understandably, these patients were highly stressed. I set out to relieve some of their suffering by what I then thought was going to be termed "stress management." I started teaching them how to slow their hearts, open their arteries and dissolve their muscle tension. In medical terminology, these activities are referred to as autonomic functions. It seemed logical to use the term autonomic regulation for it. My patients abbreviated this to autoregulation and eventually to "autoreg."

I soon realized my patients needed, and wanted, me to teach them methods for self-regulation and healing. I also recognized that self-regulation goes far beyond any ideas of autonomic regulation. I started a search for a simple term that, in practical terms, would declare my purpose.

Again, my patients solved my problem. They stayed with the term autoreg as I experimented with different words. In the end I decided to follow their lead. Looking back, my work with autoregulation evolved in the following sequence.

* *Stress management*
* *Autonomic regulation*
* *Self-regulation and healing*
* *States of consciousness*

One of the essential lessons my patients taught me is this: Slowing the heart rate, keeping the arteries open and slow, even breathing profoundly affect our mood and state of the mind. These basic methods of autoregulation are very effective in dissipating anger and anxiety even when that is not our intended purpose. But this is just a beginning. Autoregulation reveals the path of self-regulation and healing. A passage through the realms of self-regulation inevitably ushers a person to higher states of awareness and consciousness.

Autoregulation is self-regulation and healing with energy.

Autoregulation, as defined in this volume, is self-regulation and healing with energy — energy of tissues, cells and molecules. It is self-regulation with full benefits of the science and technology of modern medicine. It is self-regulation with objective, measurable, and reproducible electromagnetic, molecular, and cellular changes in our biology. It is self-regulation in which the individual practicing these methods is the true judge of their efficacy, and not some pseudo-scientist with silly notions of double-blind cross-over methods of medical research.

Autoregulation is not healing with hypnosis, psychoanalysis, psychotherapy, regression, progression or biofeedback.

Hypnosis is a valuable treatment option. Nobody ever becomes toxic with hypnosis as most people taking drugs do. The hypnotist puts the patient into a trance and puts him out of his misery. The patient obtains immediate relief though he has no understanding of how he obtained it. It is my personal observation that the good effects of hypnosis almost always wear out with time. Continued hypnosis fails to sustain the initial benefits.

Autoregulation, by contrast, is a slow process. It generally does not offer immediate relief. Most people learn autoregulation methods over days and weeks. *However, once learned, the methods of autoregulation never lose their clinical efficacy.* Indeed, the longer the person practices autoregulation, the more profound its benefits. No one ever unlearns autoregulation. Autoregulation work even when an individual is in the throes of an acute life-threatening illness, though the benefits may be rather limited under such circumstances.

The critical difference between autoregulation and hypnosis is this: Autoregulation is a path of independence. Hypnosis and the placebo effect are the paths of dependence on someone else.

THE CORTICAL AND LIMBIC STATES

In my working model of self-regulation (and healing) in

clinical medicine, I use the term "cortical state" to refer to a state of the human condition that calculates, computes, competes, cautions, creates stress, causes immune dysfunctions, and culminates in disease. I use the term "limbic state" to refer to a state of the human condition that cares and comforts, creates images of health, and allows the injured molecules, cells and tissues to heal by their own innate healing abilities.

For the *limbic condition* to heal, it must first be freed from the relentless censor of the *cortical mind*. Switching off the thinking cortical mode is simple to understand at an intellectual level, but it requires considerable practical experience in real life situations. The harder one tries not to think, the more difficult it becomes. This is almost a universal experience. Some very intuitive people turn out to experience exceptions to this.

A Body-Over-Mind Approach to Healing

We often hear about the concept of healing with a mind-over-body approach. In my own work with self-regulation, I do not find this to be sufficient for reversing chronic indolent diseases. I see superior clinical results when my patients adopt a "body-over-mind" approach, i.e., when they learn how to listen and attend to their tissues and shut out their thinking minds.

We take pride in our minds, but healing is not an intellectual function. Healing cannot be forced upon injured cells and tissues by a demanding mind. Rather, healing occurs when the tissues are set free from the ceaseless censor of the mind. My patients were unable to control their asthma and migraine attacks, lower their raised blood pressure, or reverse other chronic illnesses with a *mind-over-body* approach.

In my own clinical work, a *body-over-mind* approach has given me far superior results. Many of my patients reversed their tissue injury and chronic diseases when they learned how to *attend* to their tissues. Tissues evidently know how to respond. We need only to learn how to shut off our thinking *cortical* minds and attend *limbically* to our molecules, cells, and tissues in duress. This is not simply a clever play on words. Molecular repair and healing are visceral and *limbic functions*. Molecules, cells and tissues do respond when we attend to them.

Molecular Medicine

I defined the term molecular medicine earlier in the explanatory note. It is a practice of medicine that manages chronic health disorders without drugs but with integrated treatment protocols of environmental medicine, nutritional medicine, medicine of self-regulation and medicine of physical fitness. Drug therapies are necessary for symptom relief on a short-term basis. According to the precepts of molecular medicine, however, the concept of drugs as the true agents of change from a state of chronic disease to a state of health is fundamentally flawed.

Health, in molecular terms, is the molecular mosaic that balances the life span against the aging-oxidant molecules; disease, a state of molecular disarray in which the latter overwhelm the former. *This is where all diseases begin.*

Chapter 2

The Butterfly
and
Veteran Dieters

Some say obesity is the material of the psyche, others that it is woven into our DNA sequences; as for me, it is all in the globules of the fat cells.

I do my daily limbic exercises on a second-floor porch with a large skylight in the ceiling. The wood frame of the skylight is deep, and the glass is set high on top of it. Distant treetops show up in the lower quarter of the skylight frame, otherwise the large glass yields a wide, uninterrupted view of the open sky.

When I do my exercises, I sometimes see insects hovering around within the skylight case. They frequently hit the glass, fall several inches, and fly up again, only to hit the glass pane again. It is a mundane sight. The bugs do not seem to recognize the obvious: In order to fly up and out, they first need to fly down and in. Usually this is but a minor distraction. When I go limbic, the bugs are no longer a part of my awareness. Sometimes a bumblebee or a wasp does distract me, especially when I see them rushing into the glass time and again, tricked by the illusion of a clear passage provided by the glass. On such occasions, my thoughts sometimes drift to how often we human beings fly into *our* own skylight glass pane.

How often does our biology spring up its own molecular skylight glass pane on us? Food allergy, in my clinical experience, is the number one cause of undue fatigue. How often do people who feel tired after eating realize that their food is the real culprit? Food addiction and food allergy are flip sides of the same immunologic coin. How often does a person realize that his craving for certain foods is a symptom of withdrawal? How often is a child in the throes of molecular roller coasters (caused by rapid hypoglycemic-hyperglycemic shifts) taught to see the link between his misery and his food? How often does a chemically sensitive woman develop a sudden headache or suffer sharp mood swings when she shops in a fabric store? How often does she recognize that high concentrations of formaldehyde in the shop air is the cause of her suffering? How often is a successful business executive awakened early in the morning with chest pain, rushed to the emergency department and given many tests only to be told that he has suffered from a "slight heart attack"? How often does he see that his heart is serving his body as a "spokesorgan"? It is rebelling against not just what might have happened to it the day before, but what has been done to it by tight arteries for years. And why does his heart choose to awaken him at that ungodly hour? Because it knows — even if he does not — that when he sleeps he is not dead.

Then there are other skylight panes. There are skylights of our own making, skylights of our past experiences and skylights of our feared future suffering. How often do we hit our heads against these skylights? How often do we smash into these skylights when we want to fly? Over and over, we seek to fly up and out. But all we do is jam up against the skylight glass of our past — of past hurts, of past guilt, of past conflicts and of past failures. Some days such thoughts persist. When they do, I make a conscious attempt to sublimate my thinking into my limbic void. My exercise is more giving when it is limbic.

One day I saw the usual chorus of my entomologic

comrades. I also saw a butterfly with brilliant crimson-colored wings with yellow and green polka dots. It was too beautiful a visitor to simply ignore. I decided to extend her the courtesy of companionship. I watched her as I did my rebounding exercises. The butterfly fluttered its magnificently colored wings in a dazzling display of aerial acrobatics. It is okay to be cortical at times like that, I thought.

The intensity of the butterfly colors and an escape from the usual gray of other insects absorbed me for how long I do not know. I came around to realize that the butterfly is in the same quandary as the other insects: She wants to fly out but cannot escape the trap of illusion created by the skylight glass. What was an engaging display for me was a struggle for life for my colorful visitor. She was exhausted and frightened now, and it showed in her strained patterns of flying. She wanted to fly up and out but to do that she first had to fly down and in. This she did not seem to know.

While rebounding, I tried to gently guide the butterfly to fly low, clear the deep wood frame of the skylight, and then fly out. My persuasions appeared to frighten the poor thing even further. I wondered if I would see her dead body the way I sometimes see the dead bodies of other insects on the porch floor the next day. A sad thought. I went back to my limbic exercises.

The butterfly comes back to me as I write about the anguish of obese people and the punishing illusion of thinness created by the weight-loss programs. I reflect upon the plight of obese people. Obese people are up against their own skylight glass. They are advised by the "nutrition experts" to diet to lose weight. With dieting, they try to fly through the skylight glass.

Again and again they try, only to be hurt and deceived and disappointed. Obese people are just as perceptive and clear-headed as their thin friends. The problem is that this maladaptation of catabolism is every bit as deceptive as the skylight glass was for my butterfly.

Catabolic Maladaptation

I coined the term catabolic maladaptation to refer to an abnormal state of metabolism that causes obesity. In this state, the fat cells are bloated with toxic fats. Fat-processing enzymes in fat cells malfunction, fat-burning enzymes in muscle cells are poisoned and muscle fibers are emaciated from disuse. The metabolic efficiency of all tissues is impaired. The individual is tired. The internal ecology of the bowel is disturbed. Food and mold allergy frequently exists. Catabolic maladaptation is caused by toxins in food, injured molecules and cells, sluggish enzymes, swollen fat cells, lame muscles, altered bowel ecology, and tired tissues.

Obese people generally understand that their catabolism (breakdown) of fat is impaired. What they usually do not recognize is that the catabolism of other nutrients such as amino acids, sugars, vitamins and minerals is also defective in obesity.

The catabolic principle evolved slowly for me. For over fifteen years now, I have focused my research and clinical interests on issues of nutrition, environment and immunity. I have cared for a large number of patients with diverse chronic immune and degenerative disorders for whom our Star Wars medicine had failed, utterly and totally. In caring for these people, I limited myself to molecular protocols of nutritional medicine, environmental medicine, medicine of self-regulation and medicine of fitness. Most of my patients lost weight as they obtained symptom relief and gained higher levels of energy, even though weight loss was not our intended goal. As I observed these people suffer for long periods of time and eventually succeed, the true nature of these problems of molecular toxicity of foods, enzymatic poisoning caused by pollutants, disuse atrophy of mitochondria, catabolic insufficiency and obesity (the catabolic maladaptation) gradually took shape in my mind.

With dieting, overweight people, like my butterfly, attempt to fly through the unyielding glass of catabolic maladaptation. Like my butterfly, they get hurt each time they fly into the glass. And like my butterfly, they try again, over and over, again and again. They starve. They scream in anguish. They scheme of clever ways of fooling their toxic fat cells. They lose weight initially by losing water and muscle. They become flabby. Their fat-burning muscle fibers thin out. Their fat-burning enzymes become even more sluggish. Their cells become more fat-toxic. They begin to gain weight *even as they eat less and less.* The scarred veteran warriors of this dieting war bear testimony to their attempts to fly through their skylight glasses. Obese people need to fly up and out of their catabolic glass frame by flying around their glass. How can they understand the illusion if their "nutrition experts" do not?

Obese people, first and foremost, need to understand the catabolic illusion. They need professionals who can guide them away from dieting and away from herculean exercise programs. The catabolic illusion has several facets, and all are deceptive.

The catabolic illusion masks the molecular mimicry of catabolic maladaptation.

Nineteenth-century English naturalist Henry Walter Bates studied butterflies in the Amazon river basin during the mid-1800s. He observed how birds found certain species of butterflies to be "tasty" while they avoided other species that were "toxic" and made the birds sick. He further observed how some tasty butterflies protected themselves from birds by mimicking the appearance of toxic butterflies. This hypothesis of one species exploiting the defense system of another species is called Batesian mimicry.

Molecules mimic each other, and so do cells and tissues. Molecules mimic each other for diverse reasons. Sometimes it is beneficial for the organism, at other times it is injurious. Molecular and cellular mimicry is recognized by naturalists and biologists in nature, and by astute clinicians in the clinical practice of medicine.

What my butterfly taught me, in a way, is very similar to what Bates butterflies taught him. Mimicry is ubiquitous in biology. Bates butterflies found a way to use mimicry for preservation. My butterfly fell victim to the mimicry of her nerve cells which mistook the skylight glass for a clear passage to the open air. Obese people need to learn, understand and observe how molecular and cellular mimicry can both help and hurt. Dieting for thinness is a cruel form of molecular mimicry. It hurts the person in many ways.

First, the catabolic illusion leads the obese person to diet, eat less, and down-regulate his fat-burning enzymes when in reality he really needs to eat more and up-regulate these enzymes.

Food fuels the furnace of metabolism; exercise stokes its fire. This simple fact of human biology is widely misunderstood. The merchants of our rich dieting industry know the money is in packed frozen foods. It is not in teaching people simple facts of biology. Our TV, our magazines, our newspapers, all carry the same message: Diet and be slim. Who has the courage to go up against all this?

While the men of money in the dieting industry see their profits clearly, the professional dieting experts on their payroll have their own skylights. So do the dieting experts in our hospitals and public institutions. They scheme of clever diets. I sometimes wonder if there are any health professionals who profit more from their own incompetence than the medical "experts" in the weight-control business. Veteran dieters know this all too well. They pay for their weight loss over and over again.

There is an appalling paucity of knowledge of human biology and metabolism among our weight-control experts. Perhaps the worst offenders are those who work in our hospitals. In the chapter *Life Span Food Choices*, I give detailed lists of food choices and include my reasons for dividing foods into life span and aging-oxidant categories.

Second, the catabolic illusion pulls the obese person toward sugar-burning exercise whereas his bloated fat cells really need fat-burning exercise.

The essential nature of obesity is down-regulation of fat-burning enzymes. The real issue is how to up-regulate these enzymes and not merely burn calories.

The notion of burning calories to lose unwanted pounds of fat is pervasive in the United States. Hardly a week goes by that I do not hear someone outline his ambitious plans for exercise to burn out his excessive weight. With rare exceptions, all he gets is sore muscles, pulled tendons and bruised spirits.

Exercise that causes sweating and heavy breathing and gives us tired muscles is *sugar-burning* exercise. I call such exercise "cortical exercise." Cortical exercise is of very limited value for up-regulation of fat-burning enzymes. Up-regulation of fat-burning enzymes requires *slow, sustained* exercise. I call such exercise "limbic exercise." For reversing catabolic maladaptation, an overweight person needs to know the critical difference between these two types of exercise. I discuss this subject at length in the companion volume *The Ghoraa and Limbic Exercise.*

The health professional advising the obese person so often fails to see the critical difference between sugar-burning cortical and fat-burning limbic exercises. It is only when the catabolic illusion is dissipated with knowledge and insight that the obese person has any real chance of correcting his catabolic maladaptation for good.

Third, the catabolic illusion blinds us to the problems caused by food and mold allergy.

Food and mold allergy feed the molecular roller coasters triggered by dieting and ill-advised herculean exercises for burning off fat. Hives caused by allergy are seen by all. The internal "hives" of the bowel, the liver, the heart and other organs are not obvious to the innocent victim of the merchants of our dieting industry.

Fourth, the catabolic illusion feeds molecular roller coasters.

Sudden rises in blood sugar evoke sudden insulin responses. Bursts of insulin drive the blood sugar down to hypoglycemic levels and trigger the release of adrenaline and related chemicals. This causes apprehension, light-headedness, mood swings, heart palpitations, and other signals that call out the body's need for more quick energy. The person reaches for more sugary snacks and repeats the whole cycle of the molecular roller coaster.

Fifth, the catabolic illusion misplaces the blame of sugar, salt and fat craving on "the problems of the mind."

Salt causes, perpetuates and intensifies salt craving. Sugar feeds the sugar craving. Fats foster fat craving. All three feed upon each other. Craving is not a problem of the mind. Craving is a form of catabolic molecular mimicry.

Sixth, the catabolic illusion keeps the obese person in the dark about the fundamentals of metabolism.

Food increases basal metabolic rate (BMR), which is the essential metabolic indicator of the body's ability to generate and expend energy. Thin people have higher BMRs; they burn calories at a much faster rate than their obese friends. How can we increase the BMR? By eating more. How is the BMR lowered? By dieting.

Seventh, the catabolic illusion confounds us about the issues of the bowel ecology.

The ancients, it seems, intuitively knew the central role of the bowel in preserving health. I have had an opportunity to examine several thousand bowel biopsies. I have also cared for a very large number of patients with indolent chronic bowel disorders. This experience has led me to conclude that preservation of normal gut ecology is *essential* for promoting good health and optimal weight. I discuss this subject at length in my monograph *The Altered States of Bowel Ecology and Health Preservation.*

In altered states of bowel ecology, the bowel is starved of energy (the bowel arteries are in spasm), uneven in its rhythm (cramps, diarrhea, constipation), depleted of its digestive acid and enzymes, unable to keep undigested foods out (the so-called Leaky Bowel Syndrome), overgrown with yeast and infested with parasites. Obese people often have an altered bowel ecology. They cannot solve the problem of the catabolic maladaptation without first restoring their bowel ecology to normal.

Eighth, the catabolic illusion belittles the importance of limbic listening.

Western culture, in many ways, is a culture of confession. We seem to believe that to talk about hurt is to understand it, to find a name for a person's anguish is to define it, to intellectualize about suffering is to dissipate it, to think about disease is to heal it. My clinical work has led me to serious reservations about such simplistic notions. Again, the veteran dieters will bear testimony to the limited value of such intellectual gymnastics. In the chapter *On Limbic Eating*, I discuss the essential need to learn to listen limbiclly to our biology, to the demands of our tissues and to the *real* hunger signals.

An obese person needs to see all the illusions of the catabolic maladaptation, clearly, completely and unequivocally. He needs to see all the faces of this monster. This requires learning, eating life span foods, doing limbic exercise, observing the effects of these steps, and repeating this cycle over and over again until the catabolic maladaptation is permanently reversed.

An obese person needs to gain muscle mass and increase the amount of fat-burning tissue. That usually means a slight initial weight gain (or at least absence of weight loss). This happens because muscle tissue is heavier than fat tissue. Only then can he hope to increase his rate of burning (and losing) fat. This is the beginning of the process of the reversal of catabolic maladaptation. This is the beginning of a permanent change.

An obese person needs to learn how to fly down and in before he can fly up and out.

Obesity is a physical and a pathological state.

The obese state is a physical state. This is self-evident. We all recognize this. Obesity is not a normal state. This is also self-evident.

What is rarely realized, however, is that the *essential nature* of obesity is a profound disturbance of energy enzymes. Obesity is a pathological state, and it can be explained and understood as molecular defects. The structural and functional changes observed in the cells, tissues and organs of overweight people are consequences of molecular deviations.

Obesity is not a problem of the mind.

Ask an obese person if he has any problem thinking clearly. Next, ask him if he is confused about matters of health, energy, fatigue, or the hunger pangs that come with dieting. Then ask him if he overeats when he is angry. Next ask a thin person if he overeats when he gets angry, hostile or depressed. The probable answers will be that both obese and thin people sometimes overeat when they are angry. At other times they do not. Obese people do not have a monopoly over problems of the mind. Nor are thin people immune to eating disorders. Indeed, depressed people almost always lose weight as the depression deepens. Anti-depressants cause weight gain. There has never been a scientific study showing that obese people suffered from more anger, hostility or stress than thin people *before* they became fat. Obesity, once established, of course, brings forth its own heavy load of fatigue, anguish and stress.

Obesity is caused by injured molecules and injured cells.

Obesity is a matter of injured molecules and cells. It is a matter of toxic and oxidized fats, denatured and cross-linked proteins, disfigured and mutated sugar molecules, depleted enzymes, absent micronutrients, synthetic toxicants and poisonous heavy metals. It is a matter of trans fatty acids in margarines that our body cannot utilize, and of cyclic fatty compounds, produced during food processing and deep-frying, that are toxic to our molecules.

Injured molecules and cells need more, not less, food for healing. Dieting starves the sick molecules that yearn for nutrition and health. Dieting further injures the already damaged molecules, cells and tissues. This book is about losing weight and gaining more energy by eating more life span foods (foods that sustain our life span) and eliminating aging-oxidant foods (foods that cause premature aging).

Obesity is but one symptom of the most pervasive disorder of our time, the "dis-ease syndrome."

The dis-ease syndrome is characterized by an accelerated oxidative molecular injury. In this state, oxidative molecules of stress, toxic foods and environmental toxicants feed the furnace of molecular oxidation and cause a molecular burnout. I discuss the global issues of this syndrome in *The Cortical Monkey and Healing.* In the present volume, I will describe in detail the aspects of autoregulation that are essential for success in achieving and maintaining life span weight. Autoregulation is not mind-over-body healing. It is about perceiving the energy in our tissues, enhancing that energy, and finally directing it to specific tissues for specific results. In the companion volume, *The Ghoraa and Limbic Exercise*, I discuss strategies for a *body-over-mind* approach to slow and sustained exercise for attaining and maintaining the life span weight.

Obesity is virtually nonexistent in tribal cultures.

We often hear about the role of genetics in obesity. We are told to see how often the children of obese people are also obese. That is true. Overweight parents often have overweight children. But the issue of hereditary factors in obesity is not such a simple matter. The children of obese parents are usually exposed to the same risk factors that cause catabolic maladaptation and obesity in their parents. It is interesting to consider the incidence of obesity in tribal cultures. There is virtually no obesity among tribal cultures. Yet when these people move from tribal living to "advanced" living, obesity appears within a few decades. Eskimos in Alaska and American Indians are two unmistakable examples of this phenomenon. Obesity in both groups was almost nonexistent when they lived in their traditional ways. However, obesity and alcoholism are dominant health problems in both ethnic groups now.

Psychosomatic and somatopsychic models of disease are artifacts of our thinking.

Our diseases are burdens on our biology. These burdens are imposed upon our genetic makeup by our external and internal environments. The intensity of suffering caused by these burdens is profoundly influenced by a third element — the choices we make in our response to these burdens.

The catabolic maladaptation, the root cause of obesity, is also a consequence of environmental burdens on our genetic makeup. The genetic factors involved here, as we shall see later, are of much lesser significance than the external elements. These elements include toxic foods, molecular roller coasters caused by aging-oxidant foods, nutritional deficiencies, dysfunction of lipases (enzymes that regulate fat utilization), poisoned mitochondrial oxidative enzymes (that burn fat to generate energy), confused and bloated fat cells and tired muscle cells suffering from disuse atrophy. One of my overweight patients put it most succinctly:

"Dr. Ali, I am very fat now. I used to be very slim. I really do know my problem. My problem is simple: My metabolism has shut."

True insights in our biology, it seems to me, usually come through suffering. This person is so right. Shut metabolism! That is exactly what the catabolic maladaptation does.

A physician's most treasured teachers are his patients, and not any laboratory mice or medical students (whose services are usually "volunteered" by their professors when they use them as their experimental animals for their research projects).

Obesity cannot be reversed with dieting.

Dieting does not work. Ask any veteran dieter. In the rare event when people do *seem* to be succeeding with weight loss and show improvement in their molecular health and level of energy, they do so for reasons which have nothing to do with dieting. There is an abundance of pundits of dieting who peddle their potions as they plunder the pockets of their unsuspecting victims. This book seeks to explode the myth of dieting and the mystique of dieting pundits.

I intend to give the reader a well-structured, easy-to-follow program for attaining life span weight, keeping the muscles firm and vigorous, spurring fat-burning enzymes into brisk activity, and shedding unnecessary pounds of fat. Still, I recommend the reader find a professional who is knowledgeable in the subjects of nutrition, metabolism and the impact of environment on human biology. The clinical application of the catabolic principle should be easy to master for any professional with some experience. As for autoregulation, I recommend the books mentioned previously, and when possible, workshops on meditation and self-regulation given by professionals who are knowledgeable and experienced in those areas.

Obesity reversal for many people is a burden to be relieved only by a miracle.

This miracle, however, can be attained. But it is not a miracle that involves a secret potion or an ancient concoction or an exotic plant root from a distant land or even a triumph of modern synthetic chemistry. It is a miracle of learning, of knowledge, of catabolic insights, and of hope and life.

Chapter 3

Life Span Weight

What is life span weight?

Life span weight refers to the ideal weight that will allow an individual to live his expected life span lean, fat-free, fit, energetic and in perfect health.

Life span weight is not simply a *reduced* weight. Children and adults become emaciated in many countries during periods of famine. Starvation consumes the muscle mass before it depletes the body fat stores. Thinness achieved through starvation has disastrous effects on the long-term health of an individual, whether it is caused by a famine or drought in an impoverished country or by famine of misguided dieting in an impoverished state of mind.

A thin, muscleless frame is not a healthy frame. It is not *thinness* that we should be after. It is a *lean, fat-free and vigorous body* that gives us life span weight and a life span perspective of health and life.

The National Institutes of Health, in its 1985 consensus report, defined obesity as an excess of adipose tissue (body fat) that frequently results in significant impairment of health. As can be expected from a consensus report of nutrition "experts" who do not practice nutritional medicine, this is a statement singularly devoid of any merit. It is of no relevance to those who are serious about preventive medicine and health. First, how do we define *excess* of adipose tissue? The consensus report does not tell us that. Second, how do we know what this consensus report considers *significant impairment of health*? In classical medicine we think only of two states: a state of disease and a state of absence of disease when our CAT scans and blood tests do not allow us to select a disease label for a given patient. I have never seen a medical textbook of medicine that dares to define health. There is a third problem with this statement. In preventive medicine, we do not wish to wait until significant impairment of health has occurred before we regard a particular weight as unacceptable from a life span perspective.

Some nutrition experts consider an increase in weight of 20% (or more) over the ideal body weight as a health hazard. Again, they do not tell us what the ideal weight is. In our life span perspective, we are oriented toward optimal health with vigorous energy for the duration of our expected life span. We are not merely narrowly focused on issues of *health hazards.*

Life span weight is the specific weight for a person that gives him the best chance for living his full life span in perfect health. Good health for an individual is not what a professional can determine by consulting his computer charts and graphs. It is a weight that a person must determine by himself by limbically listening to his body tissues. A knowledgeable professional is necessary for guidance in making good food choices and for outlining optimal programs for exercise and self-regulation. Basic knowledge of human biology and energy dynamics is essential for increasing muscle mass, decreasing body fat, and achieving and maintaining life span weight. Commonly used weight tables (prepared by the Metropolitan Life Insurance Company or other sources) are also valuable as a general guide. I have included suggested guidelines at the end of this chapter. But the true determinant of what constitutes the life span weight for a person has to do with his sense of energy, vitality, fluidity of motion, and ability to enjoy his work and personal time in full health. The *key issue* here is a perspective of his life span, not simpleminded efforts to lose weight by starving his tissues. The distinction between the two is critically important.

WHAT IS HEALTH?

One of the core problems of medicine today is this: We physicians know what diseases are, but we have no concept of what *health* is. We physicians have been turned into what my friend Choua calls "disease doctors" by the prevailing mode of drug medicine. We have lost the distinction between absence of disease and the presence of health. Society pays a heavy toll when its physicians are turned into disease doctors.

What is health? This question is rarely, if ever, raised in medical schools. Whenever someone dares to talk about the holistic approach to health, he is very cautious not to be misconstrued, cautious to a degree that his message becomes a non message. His students are baffled rather than enlightened.

So what is health? Health is to open one's eyes in the morning with a heart full of gratitude for the Lifegiver. It is a profound sense of gratitude for being able to spring out of bed. I know far too many people who cannot do this simple task.

Health is to start a day with fluidity of movement of torso and limbs. In the chapter, The Ghoraa and Limbic

Running, I describe some gentle stretches for all the major muscle groups of the body with focus on the neck, back and shoulders. I recommend a liberal intake of 12 to 24 ounces of fluids at this time. (It is an excellent time to take nutrient supplements unless stomach difficulties make it necessary to take them during breakfast.) Health is limbic exercise in the morning to obliterate the cortical clutter that holds us captives. Health is a breakfast that leaves us with as much energy as it finds us with.

Health is doing a day's work with energy and limbic openness. It is a day's work done with a kind awareness of the tissues beneath our skin. It is a day's work done with a sense of fairness to those to whom our work obliges us. It is a day spent with sensitivity to people around us.

Health is finishing a day's work with as much energy as we start it with. Health is personal time with energy and an inner, visceral sense of calm. Health is going to bed at night with as much energy as we had in the morning. Health is sleeping like dead wood.

Health is two to three odorless and effortless bowel movements a day, without cramps and without bloating. The normal bowel transit time should be eight to 14 hours. This means our prevailing notion of a single bowel movement in the morning is inconsistent with the motility requirements of the bowel. This is a critically important issue. I personally will not manage any immune or degenerative disorder without first restoring the internal ecology of the bowel to a normal state. This cannot be achieved without restoring a normal bowel transit time.

Large stools, small hospitals.
Small stools, large hospitals.

The ancients seemed to have intuitively understood that most chronic diseases begin in the bowel. Dennis Burkitt reiterated this relationship in contemporary medium when he spoke of a choice for a society: It can keep its stools small and build large hospital or allow the stools to be large and build small hospitals. Human molecular defenses, it seems to me, are plants rooted in the soil of the bowel contents. I discuss this essential subject at length in my monograph *The Altered States of Bowel Ecology and Health Preservation.*

Health is personal time for personal limbic choices, for getting involved with things that help us escape the cortical tunnels of narrow focused living. Health is living in limbic openness.

Am I last on the list of my priorities?

How many of us live our lives at the bottom of the list of our priorities? How often are we aware of what passes within us, under our skins? How many of us go out and buy chocolate or a heavy cheesecake when we think of doing something for ourselves? Or go out for a heavy meal and return with a bloated stomach and a sense of emptiness in our hearts?

I must be kind to my body,
so my body can be kind to me.

Health is being kind. Kind to those around us. Kind to animals. Kind to flowers. How can we be kind to flowers? By looking at them and perceiving their beauty. And yes, health first and foremost, is being kind to ourselves. Health in its finest form is being in one's native state, just *being*.

Health is living with a purpose.

It is one thing to understand the causes of obesity and ill health. It is altogether a different matter to live a life with freedom from both. Life cannot be sustained without a purpose. Before undertaking any efforts to change our view of foods, eating patterns and physical fitness, we need to recognize a larger need for a purpose in life.

How many people learn to live with impossible odds through their efforts to sustain someone else? How many people live angry lives? Angry with people. Angry with things. Angry against things that do not exist. Nutrition is a part of the human condition and yogurt alone will not do it.

We Americans are obsessed with aging. Aging, we are told, is another name for losing. We lose hair. We lose vigor of our skin. We lose strength of our muscles. We lose sharpness of our mind.

One sure sign of aging.
Things do not matter anymore.

****

One sure way to beat the aging process.
Find something that does matter.

****

ABSENCE OF DISEASE
IS NOT ALWAYS PRESENCE OF HEALTH

I wrote the above words in *The Cortical Monkey and Healing* to discuss one of the major problems with the prevailing mode of drug medicine. Diseases, with rare exception, are not sudden departures from health. Before people become sick enough for us physicians to diagnose diseases, they go through variable periods of a dis-ease state. It is during this state of dis-ease that we have the most potential to use nutritional, environmental, self-regulatory and fitness approaches to achieve optimal health and life span weight. This is also where the biggest hurdle in the way of good health is. We physicians fail to distinguish between the presence of disease and absence of health. We are generally very uneasy with early evolving disease when the *right* numbers from our chemistry analyzers and CAT scans are not forthcoming. The subject of achieving and maintaining the life span weight cannot be separated from the larger subject of absence of health.

In the preface of this book and in the chapter, The Butterfly and Veteran Dieters, I define the term catabolic maladaptation and indicate that obesity is a visible reflection of the deeper catabolic problems included in this term. I describe in further detail aspects of this maladaptation in the chapter, On the Nature of Obesity.

The catabolic maladaptation includes all those molecular and energy events that threaten health and life span. Specifically, it includes dysfunctions that cause fat-burning muscle fibers to become emaciated, fat-burning enzymes to become sluggish, fat cells to become bloated with toxic fats, and health-preserving molecular pathways to be thrown into roller coaster highs and lows. The person feels "not healthy," tired, and depleted. He begins to add layers of fat over his thinned-out muscles. Each pound of additional fat feeds the catabolic disorder. Misguided efforts to lose fat only worsen the problem.

The catabolic regulation for maintenance of life span

weight is a molecular and cellular function, primarily located within the fat and muscle cells and *not* in the hypothalamus in the brain as our obesity experts think. In the chapter, On the Nature of Obesity, I present scientific evidence to dispel the myth that there is a hypothalamic set point for weight control and describe how molecular and cellular intelligence at the levels of fat and muscle cells determines whether we remain lean, fit and energetic or become obese, fatigued and listless.

No cell can preserve its health and integrity without a layer of healthful fats in its covering membrane. I sometimes wonder why nature would make fats in food so necessary for satiety if not to assure a healthy supply of fats for the cell membranes. The fat cell and its fat-processing enzymes *know* how many *healthy fats* it needs to store and how many unwanted fats it must burn to maintain a lean, fat-free, fit body. The muscle cell and its fat-burning enzymes *know* how much energy they need and whether they need it fast (generated by burning sugars) or whether they need it in a slow and sustained fashion (generated by burning fat). What we need to do is to understand this and respect the wishes and actions of the catabolic control.

It is not our purpose to lose weight to reach our life span weight, and in the process become thin, flabby, tired, slothful and unhealthy. Our goal should be to eat well, to attain and maintain our life span weight with more energy, less weight, better looks, improved health and longer life.

Tissues loaded with toxic fats are tired tissues. The cells in these tissues are bloated, their enzymes sluggish. The cells have diminished energy levels. They are slow in producing energy, slow in their work, slow in ridding themselves of toxic wastes, and slow in recovery from injury. Fat cells are tired cells that cannot burn fat; instead they hoard yet more fats.

Tired tissues have tired metabolism. Tired metabolism makes people tired.

I'm too short for my weight.

A short-statured patient once gave me her insight into why she was unable to lose weight. Are there people who are really too short for their weight? I do not know if she was being philosophical about the matters of weight, health and happiness. She reminded me of some French models I once saw on the left bank of the Seine in Paris. They were leggy as French models generally are. Looking at them I felt almost certain that they suffered from some eating disorders, bulimia, anorexia or perhaps both. Were they too tall for their weights?

Questions like these, even when raised in jest, help us put the subject of life span weight in proper perspective. The real issue in all such discussions should be optimal health for the full life span and not any preconceived notions of how thin or fat a person should be. A thin tall bulimic model is in no better physical form than a short plump woman who is comfortable with her life. Right food choices and slow, sustained exercise will help them both, though in different ways. The model, of course, may feel compelled to remain thin, albeit in poor general health, for professional reasons.

It is well known that obesity renders the obese person vulnerable to heart disease, high blood pressure, strokes, diabetes, degenerative disorders and many forms of cancers. According to the estimates of the National Institutes of Health, about 35 million Americans are overweight to a degree that puts their health in jeopardy. Again, I see difficulty with the Institutes' number. It has been estimated that up to one half of all Americans (over 125 million) have tried to reduce weight by dieting at one time or the other. It seems to me that people have a better sense of this problem than the experts at the National Institutes of Health.

There is a miracle.

Less weight, more energy, better health and longer life with the catabolic principle? A miracle? Yes, there is a miracle hidden in the catabolic principle. It is not the miracle of an exotic potion, an elusive nutrient, a wonder drug, a surgical skill or a more clever way of thinking about food.

The catabolic principle *is* a miracle. It is a miracle of reality, a miracle of knowledge, of insight and of results. It is a miracle of a permanent change.

WEIGHT & HEIGHT TABLE

MEN

HEIGHT	SMALL FRAME (+-3)	MED FRAME (+-5)	LARGE FRAME (+-6)
5'2"	128	132	140
5'3"	130	134	143
5'4"	132	136	145
5'5"	134	138	148
5'6"	136	141	151
5'7"	139	144	154
5'8"	141	147	158
5'9"	143	150	161
5'10"	146	153	165
5'11"	148	156	168
6"	150	159	172
6'1"	155	163	176
6'2"	158	167	180
6'3"	162	170	185
6'4"	166	175	190
RANGE	(+ - 7)	(+-8)	(+ - 12)

WEIGHT & HEIGHT TABLE

HEIGHT	WOMEN		
	SMALL FRAME (+-4)	MED FRAME (+-6)	LARGE FRAME (+-7)
4'10"	105	112	120
4'11"	106	114	123
5'	107	116	125
5'1"	110	119	128
5'2"	112	122	131
5'3"	115	125	135
5'4"	118	128	138
5'5"	121	131	142
5'6"	124	134	145
5'7"	127	137	149
5'8"	131	140	152
5'9"	133	143	155
5'10"	136	146	157
5'11"	139	149	161
6'	144	152	164
RANGE	(+-5)	(+-7)	(+-9)

Chapter 4

On the Nature of Obesity

"Weight control is a cornerstone objective for many diseases common in medicine. Substantial, prolonged weight loss is difficult to achieve. Nutrition counseling, very low calorie diets, behavior modification, exercise, intra-gastric balloon, and gastric restriction surgery are interventions that physicians may recommend patients."

The Journal of Family Practice
28:610; 1989

We physicians, in general, are ignorant of the impact of environment and toxic foods on human biology. Few things express more eloquently our intellectual bankruptcy in these matters than the advice we offer to our obese patients. Consider the above statement.

The statement starts out by recognizing that weight control is a *cornerstone objective* for many common diseases. Amen! Indeed, the list of diseases initiated, perpetuated or aggravated by obesity is extensive. It includes heart disease, high blood pressure, diabetes, arthritis, many forms of cancer, and almost *all* chronic degenerative disorders. Obesity has been correctly regarded by many as a *disease in its own right.* So it is essential for us to begin any discussion of this subject by emphasizing the central role of obesity in the causation of many diseases.

The preceding statement then moves on to recommendations that physicians may make to their obese patients. Let us consider what these recommendations might be.

NUTRITIONAL COUNSELLING BY PRACTITIONERS OF DRUG MEDICINE

The subject of nutrition counseling by physicians who regard nutritional medicine as quackery amuses me. What can the value of nutrition counseling be when it is given by people who do not believe in nutrients and who do not practice nutritional medicine? Champions of drug medicine have convinced most physicians that the only thing nutrient therapies do is to make expensive urine. That is not where it stops. Practitioners of nutritional medicine are aggressively harassed by medical boards and their licenses are threatened. I have testified for some of these physicians and I know how dirty this turf battle can be. There is the well-known case of a physician-nutritionist who was visited during his office hours by authorities with drawn guns. The authorities found some vitamin injections in his office. Vitamin bust with drawn guns! The news of this great bust was carried by the local radio and newspapers as well as some national syndicates. I met this physician at a meeting some days after this raid and asked him how he survived the event. "I lost nine pounds in three days," he replied. "Not a bad weight-loss program!" he concluded.

There are other amusing aspects of nutrition counseling

in the hands of practitioners of drug medicine. A physician colleague was concerned about his high blood cholesterol level. He consulted his cardiologist and asked if he should change his nutritional plans to lower his cholesterol level. The cardiologist told him he had a choice: He could give up many foods that he likes and live two weeks longer or he could keep eating those foods and ignore his cholesterol. The primary issue for us physicians should be the *quality* of life. This cardiologist's words come to me every time I do a pathologic examination of a leg that was amputated because the plaques in the leg arteries suffocated the tissues and caused gangrene. An appalling level of ignorance from a medical specialist! A frightening lack of sensitivity from a physician!

DIETING AND DRUG DOCTORS

Practitioners of drug medicine know dieting doesn't work. Almost all of them have referred some patients to a diet clinic and found out it doesn't work. Why do they continue to recommend *very low calorie diets?*

To our overweight patients, we physicians recommend starvation even when we know (or should know) that dieting and starvation slow down the metabolism. We do this with straight faces. How could we ever think that starvation can make the already starved, emaciated muscle fibers of obese people healthy? How could we ever think that we can starve into action the sluggish fat-burning enzymes of obese people?

How could we ever think that starvation can restore back to health fat cells that are bloated with toxic fats?

These are not hard questions to answer. We physicians in America practice drug medicine and are focused on diseases. Drugs are the tools of our trade. We have to have faith in the tools of our trade. We physicians wait for some miracle drugs that will cure obesity once and for all. Until such drugs make the scene, advice on dieting is an expedient, convenient way of dismissing the patient. We know dieting does not work, but it most assuredly saves us from an annoying problem.

Then there is another problem. The absurd notions of dieting to promote health are not fully revealed except through an understanding of the chemistry and physics of human metabolism. Chemistry and physics are subjects we physicians happily left behind in our medical schools. We are not about to return to them just to help people to lose weight. There is no money for us in the chemistry of health. Profit is in the chemistry of drugs.

BEHAVIOR MODIFICATION

When dieting does not work, we physicians recommend behavior modification. This is an interesting term. Variously, we use this term to put a cloak of scientific validity over such absurd notions as "putting the fork down between mouthfuls," "leaving some food on the plate" (why not put less food on the plate in the first place), "imagining ourselves thin while we eat," and "stepping back in the queues at the checkouts in supermarkets to kill our aggressive impulses." We ask our patients not to eat some foods, and then suggest that they reward themselves for "good behavior" by eating the foods we ask them to deny themselves in the first place. (We love to treat our patients as if they were little puppies). We offer "cognitive restructuring." I love this term. I have yet to see a patient who can relate to this term, but I love it. There are many other such pieces of clever professional advice we give our overweight patients for behavior modification.

Next, we advise our obese patients to exercise. To us, an exercise is an exercise. Most of us do not have any clear ideas about the different catabolic effects of different types of exercise. Some exercises are predominantly sugar-burning. Those exercises give our patients sore legs, sprained ankles, hyperventilating lungs, palpitating hearts and bruised egos, but no loss of fat. I call such exercises cortical exercises.

Some other exercises are predominantly fat-burning. Those exercises do not cause sweating or shortness of breath nor do they give us sore tissues. Noncompetitive and non goal-oriented, such exercises are comforting, calming and restorative. I call them limbic exercises. I give detailed descriptions of limbic and cortical exercises in the companion volume *The Ghoraa and Limbic Exercise.*

A Balloon for Mr. Moattoo

Sometimes we put balloons in the stomachs of our obese patients. Oh! the things our gullible, unsuspecting patients let us do to them. Common sense is so uncommon in our work. Years ago when I first read about stomach balloons, I imagined a conversation between an obese man and his doctor about a gastric balloon therapy; it went something like this:

"Mr. Moattoo, you have a pretty bad weight problem," Dr. Closdup says, staring into Mr. Moattoo's eyes.

"Yes, Doc," Mr. Moattoo replies with visible embarrassment.

"And our dieting program hasn't worked?"

"No, Doc. God knows I've tried," Mr. Moattoo adds apologetically.

"Mr. Moattoo, we've got to do something different. Try something new."

"Anything you say, Doc."

"There is a revolutionary new approach to this problem of obesity," Dr. Closdup says slowly, putting emphasis on every single word for Mr. Moattoo's benefit.

"What's that?" Mr. Moattoo asks, his eyes lighting up with hope.

"A gastric balloon."

"A gastric balloon? What is a gastric balloon?" Mr. Moattoo asks with surprise.

"A gastric balloon is a large balloon that I will put in your stomach to help you lose weight," Dr. Closdup answers in an authoritative tone.

"A balloon in my stomach? A large balloon in my stomach?" Mr. Moattoo repeats to himself.

"Yes, a balloon in your stomach," Dr. Closdup asserts.

"Doc, how does this thing work?" Mr. Moattoo still looks puzzled.

"The balloon in your stomach will fill it and you will not be hungry anymore."

Mr. Moattoo studies Dr. Closdup's face for a few moments, trying to determine if he is serious or if he is jesting. Dr. Closdup looks back with unblinking eyes.

"Doc, you're not serious, are you?" Mr. Moattoo asks with a disarming smile.

"Yes, I am." (Dr. Closdup allows his face to break into a slight, reassuring smile. "I attended a medical meeting last week. They said gastric balloons work very well."

"A large balloon in my stomach?"

"Yes, a large balloon to suppress your appetite. It works."

"A large balloon in my stomach?" Mr. Moattoo repeats his own words.

Mr. Moattoo's face is grim. He remains silent for a while. Dr. Closdup watches him intently, waiting for his advice to sink in. And then it happens. Mr. Moattoo's face breaks into a broad grin, as if he suddenly sees the puzzle resolve itself. He speaks with evident enthusiasm.

"Doc, I will let you put a balloon in my stomach on one condition."

"What's that?" Dr. Closdup asks with anticipation.

"I will let you put a balloon in my stomach if you first let me put a balloon in your skull. Your balloon will fill my stomach. My balloon will fill your skull. Even trade! Right?"

Patients in real life generally don't talk back to their doctors in words that can be heard. I know they do so in words that we physicians do not hear. Recently I saw a woman from what was once East Germany. She suffered from disabling fatigue, short-term memory loss and, among other symptoms, what she described as recurrent sparklike electric shocks in her head. She saw several physicians and finally was referred to a psychiatrist. "The first question this psychiatrist asked," she told me, "was if I had romance in my life. Dr. Ali, I wanted to slap that man."

TWO LESIONS THAT KILLED BUT COULDN'T BE PUT ON THE DEATH CERTIFICATE

Sometimes we recommend "gastric restriction surgery." This is an elegant bit of medical jargon. It means clamping, pleating, crumpling or simply cutting out a large part of the stomach.

Some years ago, I did an autopsy on a very obese man in his early thirties who had died two days after he had undergone "gastric restriction surgery." At the time of the autopsy, his face was disfigured, his lips swollen and dark purple, his eyes soggy with fluid, his lips contorted by a large stomach tube pulling at one corner of his mouth. His neck veins were swollen with backed up blood. His lungs were filled with fluid. His heart was flabby and bloated with fat, the heart muscle barely retaining its red-brown color. The surgical procedure had distorted the ample tissues in the dead man's body. His internal viscera, heavy with fat and stagnant blood, were difficult to dissect. Bloody tissue fluid oozed from everywhere.

Autopsy is a time for truth. Dying in earlier times was a peaceful occurrence. Our medical technology has changed that. The process of dying in modern times often leaves telling signs of its cruelty. There are times when the havoc of modern technology unnerves even the hardiest pathologists. This was a difficult autopsy for me.

"What did he die of?" The voice of the surgeon, who had performed the operation, brought me back from my thoughts of the dead and dying and modern medical technology. I hadn't noticed him as he came up on me from behind.

"He ... he died. He ... he died of .... " I cleared my throat, looking for *medically correct* words.

"What did he die of?" he repeated his question.

"He died of ... he died of fluid," I blurted.

"Fluid! Fluid in the lung, you mean," he edged me along.

"Yes, fluid in the lungs. Pulmonary edema," I said haltingly, fully aware that my words were not true to the circumstance.

"Ump! fluid in the lung! Pulmonary edema. Awful! Isn't it? I mean, the surgery went so well. And now this! Pulmonary edema kills the poor fellow. What a shame!" he said as if to dissociate himself from the tragedy.

I knew better, but kept my thoughts to myself. Young

people who die soon after surgery do not die of fluid in the lungs. This young man was no exception. Obese people tolerate surgery poorly. First, the tissues of obese people, overloaded with denatured fats, heal poorly. Second, very obese persons do poorly after surgery because their hearts are flabby with fat and cannot endure the trauma of surgery. Third, obese people find it difficult to breathe when their abdominal muscles have been widely cut open and sowed back. Most importantly, obese persons are in a state of catabolic maladaptation that weakens their molecular defenses. The young man had died of these causes. My problem was that I couldn't come up with a glib diagnostic label to explain all this to my surgeon friend. Fluid collects in the lung as a part of the dying process. Fluid was not the cause of his demise. But the phrase "fluid in the lungs" comes in handy for us pathologists when the truth is too bitter to accept.

What did this young man really die of? *He died of two "lesions."* First, there was the lesion of the young man's belief that the mechanics of Star Wars medicine would solve all of his problems. He was fat. That was a disease, and Star Wars medicine can cure all diseases. Second, there was the "lesion" of the surgeon's belief that his responsibility was trimming his patient's large stomach down to size. How did the patient's stomach get so large? How did the patient get so obese? What was the true nature of his obesity? Questions such as these are considered impertinent among surgeons who excel in "gastric restriction surgery." I couldn't engage the surgeon in such "theoretical nonsense" in the autopsy room. Nor could I put these two lesions on his death certificate. These two lesions are not included in the list of the causes of death acceptable to the American Medical Association.

Sometime ago, I asked one of my secretaries to check the page numbers of a draft of this chapter. I returned later to find that the draft was buried deep beneath a pile of files on her desk. I became curious because that was so unusual for her to do. I asked her why she did that. She told me she happened to read about the autopsy and hid the draft because she was expecting a visit from a friend. Her friend's husband was scheduled for stomach surgery for obesity. Gastric restriction surgery continues to find its unsuspecting victims.

DRUGS FOR OBESITY

The virtues of drugs used for weight loss are extolled by many physicians who regard themselves as "obesity experts." This is an area where everyone can clearly discern the essential difference between conventional obesity treatment that is recommended by obesity experts and the advice given by physicians interested in health. Drugs act by suppressing appetite; catabolic principle, by contrast, demands that the patient *limbically* listen to his appetite and never suppress it. Hungry tissues must be listened to. Hunger signals must be respected. I discuss this subject further in the chapter On Limbic Eating.

"Use of drugs for the treatment of obesity is regarded more skeptically than drug use in

other chronic diseases; this view, however, may be inappropriate ..... New approaches to drug treatment of obesity include thermogenic agents and drugs acting on the digestive system and hormones."

The Medical Clinics of North America
Jan 1989 Contents Page VIII

There are three categories of the pharmacologic effects of appetite suppressing drugs. First, these drugs stimulate the nervous system and cause many side effects. Second, appetite-suppressing drugs have several adverse effects on the heart and blood pressure. Third, such drugs increase the levels of toxic fats in tissues and lead to various degenerative diseases. Drug therapy for obesity is not only irrational, it is *unequivocally* harmful.

I have heard and read the case histories of young women and men on very low calorie diets and weight-reducing pills, who suddenly died inexplicably. What kills these unfortunate patients? Low-calorie diets impose severe molecular stresses on human biology. Appetite suppressants can cause severe molecular stresses on the heart and arteries. The likely causes of death in such cases are the combined molecular stresses imposed upon them by dieting and drugs.

So why don't drug enthusiasts see all this? This is a simple question. The simple answer is that it is much easier to give some pills and promise a miracle. It is much more difficult to listen, understand and counsel the patient. It is also the nature of this beast of drug medicine to always look to drugs for all answers.

N²D² MEDICINE

My friend Choua calls the prevailing drug-dominated medicine "N²D² medicine." The first N and D, he told me, stand for the *name of the disease* and the second for the *name of the drug*. Choua expresses it mathematically as follows:

$$\text{Name of Disease X Name of Drug} = N^2D^2$$

In N²D² medicine, Choua is fond of saying, all our work, efforts, thinking and concerns about disease start with the name of a disease and end with the name of a drug. A patient's suffering means nothing to us unless it merits the name of a disease. All methods for caring for a patient mean nothing unless there is the name of a drug associated with it. For the proponents of N²D² medicine, obesity is a disease, hence it must be treated with a drug. When Choua talks about the prevailing standards of medical practice, his favorite lines are:

Where there is a disease, there must be a bug.
Where there is a bug, there must be a drug.

"But clearly, Choua, nobody is saying obesity is caused by a bug," I remarked one day when he visited me in my office.

"Yes, that's true," Choua replied.

"Well?"

"It doesn't matter," Choua answered.

"What doesn't matter?" I asked.

Choua turned his head and looked out the window. He often does that when he does not want to answer a question.

"Why doesn't it matter, Choua!" I persisted.

"It doesn't!" Choua snapped.

"That's absurd," I said with annoyance. "What do bugs have to do with obesity?"

"There is more to this menace of N^2D^2 medicine than meets the eye," Choua spoke without looking away from the window.

"Choua, I am talking about obesity and its treatment," I protested.

"I know! I know!!" Choua answered.

"What does the menace of N^2D^2 have to do with obesity?" I persisted.

Choua was silent for a while. When Choua becomes silent in mid-thought, I know he will follow it with a diatribe. So I waited for his words to pour out.

"N^2D^2 medicine turns you physicians into drug doctors. For drug doctors, drugs are the only available tools. Your research is drug research. Your funding comes from drug companies. Your literature is drug literature. Your journals are supported by drug ads. They carry reports only of the efficacy of drugs. On rare occasions when your journals do publish an article about nondrug therapies, it is to put them down as unproven and quackery."

Choua stopped, turned his head and looked at me. I kept quiet.

"In N^2D^2 medicine, you physicians are taught how to use drugs," Choua continued after a few moments. "You are not taught how to avoid drugs. You are brought up to look to drugs for all the solutions of your problems. You pay lip service to nutrition, environment and stress control, but none of this really means anything to you. After a while, the presence or absence of a bug in the picture becomes a moot point. Drugs are the *only* way to go. All your thinking shrinks to a simple model: Where there is a disease, there must be a bug. Next, it metamorphoses to: Where there is a person, there is a bug. And eventaully, there is a drug, period! Drug-thinking drowns all rational thinking about the true causes of human suffering."

Choua stopped again but didn't turn his head.

"Choua, I know you don't like drugs, but this is absurd," I said.
"Is it? Do you really think it is absurd?" Choua's brown eyes widened.
"Com'n Choua, you are talking to someone who used to suffer from migraine attacks and unrelenting vomiting, and the only thing which put an end to his misery was demerol and ...."
"
"I know! I know!" Choua interrupted. "And I also know .... " Choua stopped himself in mid-sentence.

I understood what Choua wanted to say but didn't. My

clinical work with autoregulation was founded on my personal observations with control of migraine with limbic breathing and directed pulses. The very concept of relieving insufferable headache by things other than drugs was totally foreign to me. The very notion of ridding myself of headache with self-regulation was an anathema. That was some years ago. Then I learned how to "dissolve" my migraine with autoregulation, and went on to teach hundreds of my patients to control headache, lift themselves out of depression, abort asthma attacks, and obtain relief from severe backache without drugs and with methods of autoregulation. Along the way came some deep insights into the molecular basis of diseases and the true nature human suffering. Choua, of course, knew all that.

I looked up. Choua's large, intense eyes were fixed at me. We looked at each other in silence for several moments. Choua spoke,

"You are incarcerated in your double-blind cross-over mode of thinking. You think anything that cannot be proven with your *blessed* double-blind cross-over is not worthy of inquiry. One by one, you are turning your backs on all empirical observations made by the ancients on matters of health and disease. The ancients were intuitive people, but you can't see that with your blinders of the double-blind."

"But, Choua, surely you have to have some scientific standards in medical research," I protested.

"Scientific standards!" Choua mocked.

"Yes! Scientific standards!" I answered firmly. "How else do we know what works and what doesn't work without blinding the study?"

"You do not understand something so .... "

"Choua, you have to separate the placebo effect from the

drug effect," I persisted.

"You do not understand something so elementary," Choua ignored my comment about the placebo effect. "The combined use of several safe, nontoxic remedies gives better results in chronic diseases than one or two potent and toxic drugs. You do not understand that there are remedies that are too weak in themselves to pass your irrelevant statistical tests and yet, when combined with other nutrient and herbal therapies, *can and do* gently and slowly reverse chronic diseases.

"Do you realize what your infatuation with drugs has done to you? You have rejected all empirical observations made by men who have gone before you. You have robbed yourself of ten thousand years of man's intellectual heritage in the healing arts. You consider yourselves scientists. Science is observation. Science is not blinding yourself or anyone else.

"The only thing your double-blind does is to blind you to common sense. What common people want is health. What you seem to want is to celebrate your double-blind. You do not see the obvious: Chronic use of drugs makes people sicker with chemical consequences of drugs. People know health has something to do with nutrition, environment, stress of modern life and lack of fitness. You physicians do not know that. If you did, you would practice these arts. Your ignorant animus against natural elements blinds you to their enormous healing powers. People can tell what works and what doesn't. You physicians could also do the same before you surrendered to your drug lords. Your digoxin and your aspirin came from those observations. Don't you see it? Don't you see what your servitude to the double-blind has done? Don't you see it has made you intellectually bankrupt in matters of health and disease?"

Choua finished his monologue. His words fascinated me. I saw the truth in what he was saying but decided to say nothing. Choua looked deep into my eyes, searching for a response. There was nothing to refute. There was no challenge in my eyes. Choua walked out.

RATS, HYPOTHALAMUS AND COMMON SENSE

The dieting and drug experts of N^2D^2 medicine thrive on discussions of how the hypothalamus regulates the "set point" for body weight and body fat content. They tell us it is only a matter of time before they will develop a miracle drug which will regulate the hypothalamic set point. Once and for all, they say in voices pregnant with anticipation, the problems of obesity will be solved. A pill a day will keep all the unwanted pounds of blubber away.

How did we get so infatuated with the notions of a hypothalamic set point for obesity and a drug to regulate it for losing excess fat?

The hypothalamus is a small body of neural tissue located near the base of the brain (it is called the hypothalamus because it sits below a larger body of neural tissue called the thalamus). When a part of a rat hypothalamus called VMH (ventromedial portion of hypothalamus) is destroyed, the rat begins to overeat and becomes obese. Predictably, the fat cells of the rat fill up with fat. After gaining weight initially, the rat maintains his weight at the new higher weight (Nutr Rep Int 23:295, 1981). This was the beginning of the story of hypothalamic set point. The end of this story, the drug masters of N^2D^2 medicine maintain, will be a final solution with a new drug, another triumph of synthetic chemistry.

Further rat experiments were performed to see if the new set point (at an obese level) was indeed regulated. These experiments clearly showed that rats made obese by the destruction of their hypothalamus do not continue to eat more and become increasingly obese. Their feeding responses are not appropriate to the defense of a raised set point (*Med Clin N Am* Jan 1989 Pg 22). When this bit of medical jargon is translated into common language, it means that the so-called hypothalamic set point really does not exist. Specifically, in some experiments in which the hypothalamus of the rat had been removed and the rats were offered food that they did not like, they declined bad food and did not gain additional weight. But this does not seem to distract the set point enthusiasts. They love their set point.

The story of hypothalamic obesity is not a new story. I first encountered this subject in 1958 as a freshman medical student in my physiology class. I was taught that patients with Froehlich's syndrome become obese due to a lesion in the hypothalamus. I learned that well, not because there were a lot of kids with Froehlich's syndrome milling around the ward, but because this was a favorite question with our examiners. How often have I reviewed this subject since then? I do not remember. I did so for my licensure examination in Pakistan, in England, and in the United States, and again for my surgery and pathology board examinations.

I have never thought about this before, but as I write this now, I reflect upon the way things work in medicine. I do not remember ever seeing a case of Froehlich's syndrome in my own clinical practice, nor is it likely that I will see one soon. Since my medical school days, I have seen thousands of obese patients. I do not remember if I was ever taught the physiology and pathology of obesity in medical school or in hospital wards. I do not recall if I was ever asked any question about obesity in any of my examinations. So I wonder why my professors insisted I focus on a rare disorder that they knew I was not likely to encounter often in my professional life. Why was I never asked to focus on obesity, a health problem they knew I would see daily in my clinical work? I do not know how my teachers would answer this question. I know how I will answer this question: There is no drug money pushing the obesity "frontier." I also know this will change dramatically when the FDA approves a drug for regulating the hypothalamic set point, never mind that such a set point really does not exist. Such is the persuasive power of the drug industry. Such is the passive acceptance of the practitioners of N^2D^2.

Now some common sense. Consider the following questions.

* How does the hypothalamus regulate the weight set point of an African tribal message runner?
* How does the hypothalamus regulate the weight set point of an American couch potato?
* How does the hypothalamus regulate the weight set point of a child with food allergy?
* How does the hypothalamus regulate the weight set point of a child fed greasy hamburgers, French fries, milk shakes, soda, cereal laced with sugar, cake and candy?
* How does the hypothalamus regulate the weight set point

of people fed foods rich in pesticides?
* How does the hypothalamus regulate the weight
set point of an obese woman with down-regulated fat-
burning enzymes?

HOW DOES THE HYPOTHALAMUS TALK TO 30 BILLION FAT CELLS?

Whenever I hear about this myth of hypothalamic set point, several interesting questions arise in my mind.

How does the hypothalamus communicate with thirty billion fat cells and a similarly large number of muscle cells? This is a fascinating question. Hypothalamus enthusiasts will probably dismiss this question as irrelevant. They will say, of course, the hypothalamus sends its neurotransmitters to fat and muscle cells. Thirty billion molecules of neurotransmitters for thirty billion fat cells? And a similarly huge number of these molecules for muscle cells? And a molecule for each cell for every moment of life? And a different molecule when the person eats an ice cream cone and when he eats meat? A different molecule when he sits lazily and when he walks briskly? A different molecule for the time when he sleeps and when he runs? A different molecule when a mother cuddles her newborn and a different molecule when she screams and sprints to pull her toddler away from a speeding car? Our obesity and dieting experts are not interested in such questions.

Some hypothalamus enthusiasts will snicker at me. Doesn't this fool know the hypothalamus can send electrical impulses to the fat and muscle cells, they will taunt. They will invoke electrical impulses traveling along nerves. Now I wonder about 30 billion nerve fibers connecting 30 billion fat cells with the hypothalamus. And an equally large number of nerves connecting the hypothalamus with individual muscle fibers. And the nerve fibers have to carry different types of impulses for different types of activities. For different types of foods and activities. For different phases of metabolism. For different anabolic and catabolic needs. A preposterous proposition!

INTELLIGENCE OF THE FAT AND MUSCLE CELLS

My extensive clinical work with autoregulation has convinced me that molecules, cells and tissues have their own intelligence. They can *think*. They have the ability to respond to what is required of them, both in terms of the structural adaptation and functional responsiveness. Specifically, molecules are fully capable of "organizing" their electrons so that a certain desired structure can be attained and maintained. Function follows form. I cite an example to illustrate this phenomenon.

I have had the opportunity to care for a large number of patients who suffer from asthma. Asthma is a serious disorder. Recurrent serious illnesses and deaths from asthma are on the rise globally. Asthma, experts in drug medicine tell us, is an inflammatory lesion. The mucous lining in the bronchi, small air tubes in the lung, are swollen and stiff by inflammation and so block the movement of air in and out of the air sacs. Most pulmonologists still do not try to test and treat allergy in their patients with asthma. Of course, they believe food sensitivity has little if anything to do with it. Having so established the cause of asthma, they now recommend steroids *early* in the treatment.

I care for my asthma patients *holistically* with nutritional and environmental therapies. I also teach them autoregulation. Most of them learn to control many of their asthma attacks with autoregulation and without any drugs. How does this happen? Or, more appropriately, how *can* it happen if their bronchial tubes are made stiff and swollen by inflammation as my drug experts maintain? The answer is the muscle and mucous cells in the bronchial tube *can and do respond* when we allow them to do so. These cells are quite capable of producing molecules that counteract those that cause muscle spasm and inflammation. There are other molecules with hormonelike effects that endothelial cells (cells lining the blood vessels) secrete for such purposes. An excellent example of the latter is nitric oxide, a simple and small molecule that can perform many complex functions. I have observed clinical responses occur moments after my patients have begun to practice different methods of autoregulation. It seems that the cells and molecules in these tissues stay ready to respond.

Molecular preparedness to respond to the dynamics of life seems to be is the essence of health. I might add here that *tissues and molecules do not respond when we simply order them to do so. This is the essence of autoregulation — they know and will do what is required of them.* This has also been the single most important insight into matters of health, disease and healing during my thirty-five years of study of medicine.

Motor Molecules on the Move

Only within the past decade or so have researchers realized that the structures— sometimes called "organelles"— do not passively float from place to place within the cell but are actively transported along well laid out tracks, much the way the cars are propelled along an old-fashioned roller coaster ... Seven years ago we only had myosin, now we have at least 19 different kinesin molecules and several different dyneins."

Science 256:1758; 1992

Myosin, kinesin and dyneins are the principal motor molecules in the cell. These molecules literally "motor" the migration of the tiniest packets of enzymes that synthesize neurotransmitters and other proteins in the cells. I use the above quote from *Science* to point out how rapidly we are learning about the native intelligence of molecules and cells. This new information dispels the old notions that intelligence in the human organism is confined to the thinking cortical brain and that cells and molecules in other body tissues simply exist as materials to be deployed at the whim of the brain tissue. Indeed, a deeper look at this issue gives astounding insights into how molecules, and the electrons of which they are composed, really *live*.

Many biologists are beginning to recognize this phenomenon. In nature, there is an ongoing pattern of molecular shaping and reshaping. Electrons within atoms and molecules shift their positions to respond to their environments. I refer the reader to an excellent article on this subject by Stuart A. Kauffman of the University of Pennsylvania published in the August 1991 issue of *Scientific American*. Kauffman describes how "phase changes between solid and gaseous states can occur in *self-regulating* networks, depending on their local characteristics." He shows how thousands of genes in loops of DNA live as self-regulating networks, turning one another on and off. It fascinates me how two people working in two totally different directions can converge on the same concept. I settled on the term autoregulation from a clinical perspective. Kaufman chose the term auto-organization from his electron transfer perspective.

A butterfly fluttering in Rio de Janeiro changes the weather in Denville, New Jersey.

Many of our cherished Newtonian models of linear thinking are being challenged by the newer concepts of chaos and antichaos in physics. Chaos, in simple terms, relates to physical phenomena in which orderly, dynamic systems become disorderly. Similar initial conditions can have remarkably different outcomes. Chaos enthusiasts often dramatize their theory by the so-called butterfly effect: the notion that a butterfly fluttering in any part of the world can affect the weather in any other part. Antichaos, by contrast, is a phenomenon by which some very disordered systems spontaneously *self-regulate* themselves and auto-organize into a high degree of order.

The subjects of autoregulation, as described in this volume, and auto-organization, as described by Kaufman, are fascinating. They are also of enormous clinical importance in matters of health and disease. These subjects hold little interest for most physicians. My friend Choua thinks this is so because these ideas, and the observations based upon them, do not fit well with the precepts of N^2D^2 medicine.

THE MOLECULAR MYSTERY OF OBESITY

If there is any mystery about the cause of obesity, it is locked up in the workings of two cells: the myocyte and the adipocyte.

The myocyte (muscle cell) is the cell where the action begins and adipocyte (fat cell) is where it ends. The study of these two types of cells reveals the true nature of obesity. It is through an understanding of the structure and function of the two cells that we can begin to discern the marvels of biology that keep us lean and energetic. It is also through an understanding of these two cells that we clearly see the utter irrationality of the prevailing ideas of dieting for weight loss. Life span foods nourish these cells; aging-oxidant foods paralyze their life-sustaining enzyme systems. Fat-burning exercises energize their fat-burning enzymes; sugar-burning exercises energize their sugar-burning enzymes. Antibiotics, pesticides and fungicides destroy their enzymes as do toxic metals and industrial pollutants.

Obesity is a problem of emaciated myocytes and bloated adipocytes. Obesity is not a problem of the mind. Dieting is not a solution to the problem of obesity. Those who choose to diet do not know the biology of these cells (or do not choose to learn about these cells for reasons only they understand).

THE ADIPOCYTE

An adipocyte is a tiny cell packed with triglyceride fat. There are approximately 30 billion adipocytes in the human body. Nature designed the adipocyte as a tiny packet of stored energy. Energy is stored in an adipocyte as a tiny droplet of triglyceride fat, about 0.5 microgram in weight (A teaspoon can hold roughly 6 million micrograms of sugar). An average adult carries about 15 kg (33 pounds) of fat in his 30 billion adipocytes. Since one gram of fat contains 9 calories, it follows that an average adult has 135,000 calories stored in his adipocytes. This depot of energy can sustain an adult through a 40-50 day fast.

The term triglyceride refers to a molecule formed by three fatty acids linked together by a single molecule of a specific type of alcohol called glycerol. The types of fatty acids included in triglycerides in adipocytes reflect the composition of fatty acids in the diet. Life span foods fill the adipocytes with unspoiled, unoxidized fatty acids; aging-oxidant foods lead to the storage of oxidized fatty acids. Studies have shown that diets rich in life span oils such as oleic acid (olive oil is an important source of this oil) lead to a higher quantity of healthful fatty acids in adipocytes.

THE CELLULAR INTELLIGENCE OF THE FAT CELL

The fat cell is an intelligent cell. The wisdom of this cell shows itself in how it orchestrates the workings of the molecules that reside on its surface and those that live within it. There are molecules on its surface that it uses as hooks. It literally fishes for molecules it needs from the soup of life fluids that bathes its surface. These molecules include various hormones and other important "intelligence" molecules of the body. It has its own enzymes, and it has messenger RNA molecules that it uses to make daughter enzyme molecules.

The cell membrane of the fat cell is a marvel of biology.

*   It separates internal order from external disorder.
*   It serves as the principal clearing house for the cellular intelligence data.
*   It transforms intelligence data into physical energy and molecular changes.
*   It keeps under surveillance the intrinsic cellular self-destruct mechanisms.

* It alters its own image and structure to respond to changes in its environments.
* It serves the cell as its skin, its bowel, its kidneys, its lungs, all rolled in one.
* It influences the regulatory mechanisms for cellular growth, differentiation and reproductive potential.
* In essence, it *thinks* for the cell.

The adipocyte watches out for dangers. It fends for itself. It has sentinel molecules. It has gatekeeper molecules. It has builder molecules and scavenger molecules. It has molecules which it is willing to sacrifice and others which it guards with its life. It has slave molecules and master molecules. It has spies and messengers. The adipocyte has clear ideas of its internal organization, and it is capable of responding and adapting to preserve that order.

CELLULITE: THE GRAVEYARD OF DEAD FAT CELLS

There is an absolute limit to how much any cell can suffer. And so it is with fat cells. When toxic cyclic and trans fatty acids and fat peroxides coat a fat cell, the cell suffocates and slowly dies. Why does it happen? It happens because the cell cannot breathe through the plastic layer of these denatured fats on its surface membrane. The molecules it needs cannot come in. The molecules it wants to rid itself of cannot go out. The molecular menagerie of the cell, the ever-changing kaleidoscope of life, comes to a standstill. The fat cell dies.

Then another cell dies, and then another. The dead bodies of
these cells coalesce to form the chunks of dead fat we call
cellulite. Think of dying and dead fat cells next time you see a
child being fed french fries soaked with toxic oils and a greasy
hamburger cooked with toxic fats. And then think of what
dieting can do to the graveyards of dead fat cells. Dead fat cells
in the body cannot be brought back to life by starving the whole
body with dieting. Next, look at the label of the frozen foods
that dieting experts package for you. Denatured, oxidized oils
are not hard to spot. One clue: Almost all cholesterol-free items
in these foods are made with processed oils contaminated with
toxic fats. So stay away from cholesterol-free fats.

LIPASE:
THE SENTINEL MOLECULE OF THE FAT CELL

Lipase is an enzyme of the fatty tissues. In the fat cell,
lipase gauges the fat reserves and senses the need for bringing
in more fatty acids or putting out more fats. In the capillaries
(tiny blood vessels), lipase keeps a sharp eye out for the fat
globules that float by. Unlike many of us who indulge in Sunday
brunches in choice restaurants, lipase takes only what it knows
the cell needs. It breaks up (hydrolyzes) triglycerides in the
circulating blood into free fatty acids and glycerol molecules.
Fatty acids are pulled into the fat cell for synthesis of the
triglycerides as described above.

Human fat cells can make free fatty acids from certain

sugars called hexoses, so named because they contain six carbon atoms. These cells can make fatty acids from proteins, though molecular pathways for this are indirect and complex. But the fat cell does not prefer these molecular maneuvers. There is no molecular economy in this. The fat cell likes to keep things simple. It prefers its free fatty acids fresh, uninjured and nontoxic. It sends out the lipase molecules to harvest fresh free fatty acids much like our ancestors used to send their children to their vegetable patches at cooking time.

"We conclude that weight loss in very obese subjects leads to the increased activity and expression of lipoprotein lipase, thereby potentially enhancing lipid storage and making further weight loss more difficult."

N Eng J Med 322:1051; 1990

Translation: Our enzymes are too clever for our silly notions of dieting. Dieting is doomed to failure. When we simplistically eat less food with dieting to lose weight, the molecular wisdom of lipases in the fat cell senses an impending famine. It *knows* that deliberate attempts are being made to starve the cell it lives in. It *knows* its responsibility. It recognizes it must prepare for a famine. It sees the utter necessity for building up the reserves of the fat cells. It begins its work to hoard fat.

The fat cell also has its own cellular wisdom. What does it do? It sends out its porters (lipase enzyme molecules) to transport in more fats for what it perceives as harder times. The fat cell also has a plan B. Afraid that its porters may be sidetracked, it spawns a whole new generation of fatty acid porters by firing up its lipoprotein lipase RNA messenger. Still insecure, the fat cell has a plan C. It engages in intense motivational seminars for its young porters. The fat cells know how to guard themselves against the folly of dieting.

"Try something else," the lipases mock the dieting experts.

FATTY ACIDS TURNOVER IN THE FAT CELLS

I list below some of the important buildup (anabolic) and breakdown (catabolic) aspects of fatty acid metabolism in the fat cell.

* Free fatty acids are released from the circulating triglycerides in the capillaries by lipase enzymes.
* Free fatty acids are linked to glycerol in the adipocyte (a process called esterification) to form triglycerides.
* Free fatty acids are released from triglycerides by the catabolic (breakdown) activity of lipases within the adipocyte in a process called lipolysis.
* Free fatty acids released from triglycerides cannot be recombined with glycerol molecules that have been once used for the process of esterification.
* Free fatty acids are combined with a sugar-derived molecule called alpha-glycerophosphate.

* Free fatty acids are kept in abundant supply in the adipocyte for use as metabolic fuel.
* Free fatty acid metabolism including generation, utilization for the synthesis of triglycerides, and rerelease as metabolic fuel is governed by several families of molecules including insulin, growth hormone, glucagon (a hormone that counterbalances insulin), and receptors for the sympathetic nervous system.

The adipocyte is a versatile cell. Within its walls is a whole universe of intelligent molecules. I include above a brief listing of molecular events that occur within it, every moment of its life. The adipocyte is not a dumb glob of fat waiting to turn rancid as the obesity experts want us to believe. It is a living cell, it breathes, it observes what is around it, it responds. The adipocyte controls its own destiny, and that, of course, holds only as long as it is not poisoned with oxidized, denatured and toxic fats. Margarines kill it. So do hydrogenated oils such as oils that soak French fries when they are cooked in oils heated two to three hundred degrees centigrade for long hours. These toxic fats form a thin layer around the fat cells and literally choke the cell to death.

The preceding is a partial listing of the chemical events that occur within the adipocyte. These events govern how the cell fills up with fats and how it utilizes some of them. They show how sugars are changed into fats. They reveal how insulin and related hormones assist in the removal and storage of fats from these cells. They divulge how the adipocyte responds to electrical impulses in the sympathetic nervous system.

THE MYOCYTE

The myocyte, the muscle cell, is the mover cell of the body. It is dedicated to the single purpose of converting chemical bond energy into mechanical energy for muscle contraction and movement. This cell is a fascinating example of adaptation of cellular structure to cellular function.

The myocyte is a swinger molecule. It is long and has tapering ends, somewhat like an eel in the ocean. The soup within its walls is called sarcoplasm. Sarcoplasm, like the innards of a fat cell, is a universe unto itself. It has tiny sausage-shaped structures called mitochondria. It has tiny bags called ribosomes that make proteins. It has some dollhouses which we call Golgi apparatus.

The myocyte has two principal functional protein molecules: myosin and actin. The myosin molecule looks like a tadpole and is the quieter of the two. The actin molecule is more playful. It curls up like a snail when the muscle contracts and stretches out like a French model on a beach when the muscle relaxes. Myosin molecules make up what are called thick filaments in the muscle cells and the actin form slimmer filaments called thin filaments. The muscle contraction (shortening of myocytes) occurs by the sliding of thin filaments between the thick filaments.

Slow-twitch and Fast-twitch Fibers

The myocytes are of two types: Type I and Type II fibers. Why did nature design two different types of muscle fibers? It is an important question that gives us important insights into the inner working of the muscle cell and the subjects of obesity and weight loss.

Type I fibers are also called the "red fibers." These fibers are very rich in mitochondria, muscle protein myoglobin, and oxidative enzymes. These fibers do not tire easily and have been dubbed "fatigue resistant" and "slow twitch." One could speculate that these fibers were designed to be fatigue resistant because they were intended to maintain general muscle tone and body posture. This, indeed, is what they do. If it were not so, simple sitting on a chair or lying on the bed would cause fatigue. People who suffer from the so-called chronic fatigue syndrome do in fact become fatigued even when they sit up in a chair because their Type I fibers have been injured and cannot function well.

The second type of muscle fibers, the Type II fibers, are called "white fibers." These muscle fibers tire easily and are called "quick twitch" fibers. The Type II fibers contain a smaller number of mitochondria and have a low oxidative metabolic capacity. These fibers are mainly used for muscle activity that requires quick bursts of energy output as in sprinting and lifting heavy objects. I discuss this subject at length in the companion volume *The Ghoraa and Limbic Exercise.*

Muscle contraction is an electrochemical event triggered

by the release of a neurotransmitter called acetylcholine. A myocyte at rest is a polarized cell with a net negative electrical charge at its surface. This means that the myocyte exterior is charged positively compared to its interior. This difference in the electrical charge is maintained by differences in the concentration of certain minerals between the cell sap (the intracellular fluid) and the fluid that bathes the outside of the cell (the extracellular fluid). For instance, potassium levels are much higher in the cell sap, and sodium levels are higher in the extracellular fluid. Release of neurotransmitter acetylcholine opens certain channels in the cell membrane that permit free flow of minerals across the membrane. Changes in the concentration of potassium and sodium cause the release of calcium that activates ATPase enzyme that, in turn, makes energy available for muscle contraction.

Some types of muscle activity are predominantly fat-burning (lipolytic, in scientific jargon, and limbic, in our autoregulation terminology) while other types are mostly sugar-burning (glycolytic, in scientific language, and cortical, in our lingo). Again, I discuss these essential aspects of muscle physiology fully in the companion volume *The Ghoraa and Limbic Exercise.*

THE MIGHTY MITOCHONDRIA

Mitochondria are tiny sausage-shaped bits of tissue that float in the cell sap. There are a zillion of these tiny powerhouses in the body. As sources of cellular energy, mitochondria were recognized almost one hundred years ago. In the past, these cellular organelles were of interest only to the students of biology. The pandemic of the chronic fatigue syndrome, it seems to me, will change this. People who suffer from persistent and disabling fatigue are not interested in one more diagnostic label from their physicians. They want a deeper understanding of this problem. Some of my colleagues are waiting for wonder drugs that will cure this syndrome. My clinical experience with this problem leads me to think otherwise. It is only through a clear understanding that we can reverse chronic fatigue and restore health. I discuss this subject in detail in the companion volume *The Canary and Chronic Fatigue.*

Mitochondria are present in all eukaryotic cells (all living cells except bacteria, viruses and blue-green algae, none of which contains any nuclei), and play a central role in sustaining aerobic (oxygen-dependent) cellular energy functions.

MITOCHONDRIA: THE ENERGY CAPSULES

Mitochondria look and function like "tiny energy capsules." These energy capsules have an inner core substance (matrix) and two coverings (membranes). The outer membrane is smooth in surface, is about 50% lipids and carries specific enzymes including monoamine oxidase enzymes that oxidize and degrade stress hormones (adrenaline and related catecholamines and other molecules such as lactic acid). Anxiety and panic molecules, I might add, are predominantly the same. The inner membrane of mitochondria is about 20% lipid and 80% protein. It has folds called *cristae* and carries ATPase, which is the principal energy enzyme, and cytochrome enzymes, which are the principal enzymes involved in detoxification. The major cytochrome enzymes are designated as cytochrome P-450 enzymes and are named b, c, c1, a, a3 enzymes.

The matrix of mitochondria carries most of the respiratory enzymes of the citric acid cycle that are involved in the breakdown of sugars, proteins and fats for energy generation.

Cells that require the most energy contain the most energy generating mitochondria. The cells of the brain, the skeletal muscle and heart muscle, and the eye contain the highest number of mitochondria (as many as 10,000 per cell) while the skin cells, which do not require much energy, contain only a few hundred of them.

ATP: THE ENERGY MOLECULE

The principal energy molecule in the human body is adenosine triphosphate (ATP).

ATP molecules are produced in the cells by the oxidation of carbohydrates, proteins and fats. The enzyme systems involved in this process are collectively called cellular respiratory and oxidative phosphorylation systems. These enzyme systems are contained in the mitochondria. The energy carried by ATP molecules is used or stored depending on the needs of the body. These processes are regulated by several factors including the efficiency of enzymes, the extent of enzyme inactivation by intracellular enzyme poisons and the metabolic needs of the cells at the time.

NATURE AT ITS SUBLIME
MAN AT HIS MOST RIDICULOUS

Nature is at its sublime when we reflect on mitochondria. Man is at his most ridiculous when I reflect on chronic fatigue syndrome.

Mitochondria control their own destiny. Nature, it seems, planned to preserve mitochondria even when the cell that houses them incurs serious damage. How did nature choose to create special protection for mitochondria? It gave them their own DNA that controls their structure, function and survival. It has been estimated that approximately one trillion cells and over a quadrillion mitochondria replicate every few weeks. It is easy to see the enormous potential for errors in formation of mitochondria. Indeed, mutations involving mitochondria indeed occur with high frequency. Normally, such mutations do not cause significant energy disorder and fatigue. Such is the state of perfection endowed to mitochondria by nature.

Enter man at his most ridiculous. We have brought upon ourselves chemical and electromagnetic avalanches. We have polluted our air. We have poisoned our water. We have contaminated our food with pesticides and fungicides. We stuff the guts of our babies with antibiotics before they have any chance of developing strong bowel ecology. I reiterate here what I wrote before: Human molecular defenses exist as plants rooted in the soil of the bowel contents. Antibiotics are designer killer molecules, and so are pesticides. These are powerful oxidant molecules. earth's atmosphere is basically an oxidant environment. With our synthetic chemicals, we have enormously increased the oxidant potential of earth's atmosphere.

Poor darlings, our mitochondria! They are no match for man's ingenuity and capacity for destruction.

INJURED MITOCHONDRIA CAUSE CHRONIC FATIGUE

I consider this the essence of the pervasive problem of chronic fatigue. The injured mitochondria mutate at much higher rates. Damaged mitochondria are exhausted mitochondria. Exhausted mitochondria cannot produce sufficient ATP molecules. An insufficient supply of ATP molecules means insufficient energy. Insufficient molecular energy means clinical chronic fatigue. Chronic fatigue syndrome is nothing but a diagnostic label that we physicians love to invent to hide our ignorance. This also explains my opinion that there will never be a drug answer to chronic fatigue. The true answer is in restoring mitochondrial health, with nutrients, with environmental control and environmental therapies, with self-regulation and with physical fitness.

THE STATE OF CHRONIC FATIGUE IS A STATE OF ACCELERATED OXIDATIVE MOLECULAR INJURY

My colleagues and I are conducting several research studies with our patients who suffer disabling chronic fatigue. In one series of consecutive one hundred patients, we found mold allergy caused by IgE antibodies in all cases. About 80% of patients gave histories of extensive antibiotic therapy. About one quarter of them had elevated blood levels of toxic metals such as aluminum, mercury, lead, nickel and others. Many subjects in this study suffered from unusual degrees of stress *before* they developed a state of chronic fatigue. Viral and bacterial infections in most cases seemed to play only contributory roles. Most of our patients respond well to our nondrug nutritional, environmental and other therapies and are able to regain most of their energy. The exceptions to this are some patients with devastating chemical sensitivity, very high levels of stress arising from extenuating personal life circumstances, and very high blood levels of antibodies to Epstein Barr virus and some other viruses. Our treatment protocols, of course, are directed to reducing or eliminating the oxidative molecular stress in the chronic fatigue state. My fairly extensive clinical and research experience with chronic fatigue leads me to conclude that it is a state of accelerated oxidative molecular injury.

WAITING FOR GODOT

Now let's see what the experts of N^2D^2 medicine think about this problem.

The N^2D^2 experts at the Centers for Disease Control in Atlanta, a government agency, have decreed that the chronic fatigue syndrome must never be diagnosed if there exists an organic or psychiatric disorder that can explain chronic fatigue. The government experts often demonstrate a rare streak for making frivolous propositions. This one gets my award.

Consider their proposal: They vehemently exclude from their chronic fatigue syndrome all organic and psychiatric causes. It is as silly as saying that chronic fatigue syndrome should not be diagnosed when fatigue is experienced either by males or by females. Or when the treating physician is a male and when she is a female. Or when the sufferer has dark skin and when he has light skin. Or that this syndrome should be reserved for fatigue that is experienced when the sun is neither up nor down. If fatigue in their blessed chronic fatigue syndrome cannot be attributed to organic or psychiatric disorders, I ask, what else is there to cause fatigue?

The CDC's definition for chronic fatigue syndrome, my

friend Choua believes, is custom-tailored for men of N²D² medicine. It totally absolves them from any need to search for the cause of this "syndrome." They are quite clear in their heads. They have named the syndrome. That means they now understand the problem. That also means all that is needed now is for some drug company to come up with a drug to cure this fell disorder. Waiting for another triumph of synthetic chemistry. *Waiting for a miracle drug! Waiting for Godot!*

Watch Out, You're Becoming a Quack

Choua came over one day. He picked up a draft of this chapter and read some paragraphs about mitochondrial health and injury. He finished reading, turned his head toward the window and looked out. I watched him in silence. After a long pause, he said, "You have to be careful."

"Careful about what, Choua?" I asked.

"Be careful! That's all."

"Careful about what?" I repeated my question.

"Just be careful! You are very gullible."

"Com'n Choua, what's on your mind? Say it!" I said with mild annoyance.

"Just be careful. You know what they do to them."

"Do what to whom?" I said in frustration.

"Quacks — you know what they do to quacks," Choua looked into my eyes.

"Choua, you talk in circles. I talk about mitochondrial health. You talk about quacks."

"Just be careful, that's all," Choua repeated.

"Choua, you are too much."

"You don't understand, do you?"

"No, I don't. And if you keep talking in circles, I never will."

"You really don't understand," Choua's face softened. "This is quackery."

"Quackery!"

"Yes, quackery!!"

"Talking about mitochondria is quackery?" I was incredulous.

"Nutritional medicine is quackery. Environmental medicine is quackery. And self-regulation is quackery. Don't you see all your solutions to notions of mitochondrial health are quackery?"

Now I understood what Choua was leading to all along. I do understand this problem. The battles among physicians for territorial imperatives are often no less brutal than those between rams when the ewes are in heat.

"So?" I teased Choua.

"So if you are not careful, they'll do you in." Choua turned his head and stared at me.

"Careful about what?"

"Be careful! They will do you in good." Choua looked worried.

"They will do me in for writing about nutrition?" I pressed.

"Watch out, they don't take kindly to quacks." Choua spoke almost in a whisper.

"And they will do me in for writing about the environment?" I was beginning to enjoy Choua's worried looks.

"These things do happen."

"And they will do me in for writing about self-regulation?" I went on.

"I know you know," Choua looked away and out the window again. "You know it is not about nutrition or about environment or about self-regulation. It's about drugs. It's about money. I hope for your sake your books are not read by too many people." Choua backed away from the window and walked out.

AN INSIGHT FROM NATURE

Some evolutionary perspectives provide further insights into the role of mitochondria in health and disease.

Professor Lynn Margulis of the University of Massachusetts at Amherst first proposed in 1965 that cellular bodies such as mitochondria and plastids evolved from bacteria and algae that were long ago incorporated into cells. Unicellular organisms that existed during the early periods of planet earth (proto-eukaryotes) were sustained by a largely oxygen-free atmosphere that contained hydrogen, methane and some other gases. When blue algae learned to turn sunlight into chemical bond energy for the food chain, it released into the atmosphere large quantities of oxygen that threatened the survival of proto-eukaryotes. A marvel of biology evolved to save these organisms from the growing threat of oxygen. Bacteria-like organisms (prokaryotes) evolved that used atmospheric oxygen to make their own ATP. Recent research has uncovered clear evidence that these oxygen-utilizing prokaryotes migrated into the bodies of the threatened species of proto-eukaryotes. The microscopic invaders eventually evolved into oxygen-loving, energy-generating mitochondria. This was nature at its best. Proto-eukaryotes facing extinction from oxygen toxicity were saved by oxygen-loving prokaryotes. Proto-eukaryotes provided a home for eukaryotes; eukaryotes, in turn, detoxified the poison (oxygen) that was killing proto-eukaryotes from within. (*Science News* 252: 378; 1991)

Mitochondria evolved to save the early forms of life from death from the then aging-oxidant external element of oxygen. Now, new aging-oxidant external elements (toxic foods, industrial pollutants) are posing new threats to our survival.

MITOCHONDRIAL FATIGUE
AND MINERAL-DEPLETED CELLS

Magnesium and calcium stabilize the myocyte cell membrane and play a critical role in all energy events occurring in the myocyte. Sodium, potassium, calcium and magnesium are all life span minerals and are of great interest to us in our understanding of the problems of molecular and cellular health, fatigue, weight gain and the development of catabolic maladaptation. Mitochondrial fatigue is caused by many factors.

The principal threats posed to mitochondrial health

today arise from highly processed foods, residual toxins in foods, environmental toxicants, molecular roller coasters triggered by bad eating habits and stress molecules. Mitochondrial fatigue is also caused by physical inactivity.

Supermarket food is making us Americans sodium toxic. It is also making us magnesium deficient and potassium poor. Common use of diuretics compounds these problems. These biochemical changes provide the scientific basis for the use of liberal magnesium and potassium supplementation in the clinical management of patients with obesity and fatigue with nondrug treatment protocols of molecular medicine.

Some brief comments about calcium, a closely related mineral, may be included here. The primary problem concerning calcium is that of maldistribution. Calcium is deposited in soft tissues and blood vessels where it does not belong, and it is not delivered to bones where it is needed. Calcium in arterial plaques destroys the elastic tissue of the vessel wall, inactivates the intracellular enzymes, and leads to blockages that suffocate our tissues and give us heart attacks and strokes. Calcium in ligaments and joint capsules robs us of the fluidity of motion and gives us painful joints. Lack of calcium in bones gives us osteoporosis.

THE MYOCYTE KNOWS
SO DOES THE ADIPOCYTE

Cells are perfectly capable of autoregulation.

The cells *know*. The myocyte knows what is required of it — quick bursts of energy for pumping iron or slow and sustained energy for limbic running activity. The fat cell also knows what is required of it when it is being threatened with starvation (by dieting) or when a person responds naturally and effortlessly to subtle hunger signals, with intelligent choices of life span foods. The fat cell becomes confused when it is loaded with toxic fats. Nature didn't prepare it for such lethal assaults.

The fat cell is an intelligent cell. It senses well the

changes in the fluid that bathes it from outside, and it perceives well the changes that occur within it. Consider what happens when a fat cell is left to its own designs in a culture medium.

If the hypothalamic theory of obesity (the so-called hypothalamic set point) is valid, how does the hypothalamus send information to some 30 billion fat cells and to a similarly large number of muscle cells? By electrical impulses running through the nerves? There are not enough nerves available in our body to do this. The hypothalamus, we are told, also controls many other body organ functions. If we are to accept this interpretation, then the hypothalamus needs to communicate with trillions more cells and would require trillions of other nerves to communicate with these cells located in the other body organs.

There is another theory of obesity: The Autonomic Nervous System Theory (Diabetologia 20:366; 1981). This theory proposes that both parts of the autonomic nervous system (the sympathetic and the parasympathetic nervous systems) are involved in the development of obesity. The evidence given in support of this theory goes as follows: 1) sympathetic activity is reduced in obese subjects; 2) in animal experiments, sympathetic activity correlates inversely with food intake, i.e., when sympathetic activity is high, animals eat less and vice versa); and 3) sympathetic activity is decreased when food intake is increased with various experimental maneuvers. All such studies provide us with valuable insights into myriad molecular relationships that influence, directly or indirectly, the function of the adipocyte and the myocyte. However, it is important to recognize that all such studies represent but small facets of the ever-changing molecular kaleidoscope of biology. There are not enough sympathetic nerve fibers to innervate individual adipocyte and myocyte cells. In our broad holistic perspectives of health and disease, studies with mice and medical students must be accepted as valuable, albeit incomplete, looks at the larger problem of catabolic maladaptation.

How else can the hypothalamus communicate with fat and muscle cells? Through neurotransmitter hormone molecules? There are not enough hormone molecules to go around for this purpose either. I sometimes think about the mathematical requirements for the individual nerve fibers and for the individual hormone or neurotransmitter molecules with which the proponents of the hypothalamic theory have to contend. Trillions of molecules would be required each time a person eats a greasy hamburger. And trillions of different molecules each time he or she eats a healthy bowl of lentil soup and squash meal. Or a trillion nerve fibers to communicate with individual myocytes and adipocytes when he chooses to lift weights for 15 minutes. And a different trillion nerve fibers if he decides to run for half an hour. I wonder if our hypothalamic experts ever think of such things.

The fat cell does extremely well when it is removed from the body and grown in a tissue culture. Evidently there is no hypothalamus to regulate it in the tissue culture. There are no nerves carrying commands from an absent hypothalamus. There are no neurotransmitters, no hormones. The fat cell under these conditions autoregulates and does so very well. Recent research has shown that the fat cell in culture can produce several hormones, hormonelike substances and proteins that were previously thought to be produced only by some glandular organs. These hormones and proteins include insulinlike growth factor, apolipoprotein E (a substance that transports and regulates other functions of fats), angiotensinogen (a hormone precursor that can lead to high blood pressure), and many other proteins. Adipsin is one such protein. Low levels of this protein have been observed in some genetic types of obesity in rodents.

The fat cells in the body develop from a precursor cell. The ability of these cells to grow in response to various stimulants and differentiate (develop specific structural and functional characteristics) has been studied in both lean and obese subjects. In some studies, such adipocyte precursor cells derived from obese subjects were reported to grow at much faster rates than those from lean subjects. Is this a case of injured and confused cells that continue to make errors even when they are freed from their unhealthy environments? Based upon the observations made with other types of cells in cell cultures, I have a strong suspicion that these cells, given adequate time, will recover from their injuries and resume their normal functions.

The intelligence of fat cells and their capacity for autoregulation becomes even more fascinating when we study their mRNA species — molecules that are involved with the control and regulation of adipocyte growth and cellular renewal.

Returning to the subject of the hypothalamic set point for obesity, I ask my colleagues not to despair. For their selection, I offer a menu of set points. There may be the set points of catabolic efficiency of mitochondrial enzymes in the muscle cell that burn fat, and the set points of lipase enzymes of the fat cells that process fats in circulating blood, and the set points of metabolic pathways that try to rid the body of toxic foods and environmental pollutants. There is this problem though: These set points cannot be changed with drugs, or balloons in the stomach, or with frozen liquid diets. These set points can be changed by eating life span foods, by avoiding aging-oxidant molecules, and by rebuilding muscle mass and enzyme efficiency.

"Quack! Quack!" I thought I heard Choua mock me. I looked back. He wasn't around.

GENETICS AND HEREDITY

"But as for myself, I'd happily support the project and regard it as an unqualified success if the genetic cartographers would promise to identify nothing more than those genes governing weight. That way, perhaps, those of us destined for middle-aged spread could be genetically altered to remain eternally slim and trim without the need to devote hours of valuable sleeping, eating, drinking time to things like jogging, pumping iron, and quaffing bottles of those ghastly diet sodas."

John L. Casti in *Searching for Certainty*
William Morrow and Company, Inc. New York 1990

Mr. Casti, a mathematician of some renown, obviously wrote the above lines tongue-in-cheek. But I know of physicians who express the same thought in earnest. Sometimes they talk about the *right* weight pill that will do the trick. There will be obesity no more. Another triumph of the prescription pad. Such is the currency of silly notions among the practitioners of N^2D^2 medicine.

When molecular biologists have *perfected* the means for altering the genes that encode weight regulation, I for one will unequivocally and categorically reject their offers to change my genetic makeup. It's not that I doubt their skills in cross-breeding genes, it's just that crossbred genes usually deliver much more than what they are intended to deliver. The recipients of crossbred genes almost always get more than they bargained for. To splice genes, we first have to rupture the DNA molecule. When we rupture a DNA molecule of interest to us, we never know what other DNA molecules responsible for preserving health we have ruptured at the same time. We cannot sew them back, especially when we don't even recognize we have injured them. Years of anguish follow after our whiz kids in medicine are through with their little gene games. So I will say, "No, thank you" to these whiz kids of genetic engineering.

Sometimes I hear my colleagues point to obese children of obese parents as evidence that obesity is a genetic problem. I find that amusing. What is hereditary is the infliction of the risk factors of catabolic maladaptation by parents to their children. What is hereditary here is aging-oxidant foods on the table, pernicious ways of eating, absence of fat-burning exercises and the cruel molecular mimicry of catabolic maladaptation. For each extra avoidable pound in weight, the child carries with it the unavoidable molecular punishment of bloated fat cells, weakened muscle fibers, insulin resistance and insulin overshoot, and tired fat-burning enzymes. Each unnecessary pound in weight brings along its own *biologically* necessary baggage. This is the true nature of the hereditary burden for obese children brought up in the homes of obese parents. Uncommon hormonal and metabolic disorders are, of course, exceptions to this general order of things in biology.

When the tribal peoples from Africa and Asia emigrate to the United States, within a period of several years many of them become obese. This simple observation speaks more eloquently than all our elegant studies of DNA and RNA structure and function. It makes the most telling statement about the true role of genetic makeup in the causation and maintenance of obesity.

... we reported a total transmissible variance across generations of about 35 per cent but a genetic effect of only 5 per cent.

Genetic Factors in Obesity Pg 72
The Medical Clinics of North America Jan 1989

So that's it. The best our geneticist friends can come up with is a meager 5%. But are they right even in this?

FAT TOPOGRAPHY: FATTY LUMPS AND BUMPS

The term fat topography refers to the amount and distribution of fat in the various body organs. Specifically, this term covers two aspects of body fats: 1) the number and size of fat cells; and 2) the distribution of fat in various body organs.

The term hypertrophic obesity is used to refer to obesity associated with predominantly enlarged fat cells. The term hyperplastic obesity refers to obesity predominantly associated with an increase in the number of fat cells. The clinical relevance of these two terms, if any, is not known at the present.

Fat Genotype: The Hidden Plan for Body Fat

The term fat genotype refers to the genetic coding for the number and size of fat cells as well as for different patterns of fat deposition in different body organs. This is a theoretical concept as of now because the location and arrangement of genes that encode this information has not been determined yet. Thus, the fat genotype is hidden information. The term fat phenotype, by contrast, refers to fat that can be seen. It gives us patterns of the structure and number of fat cells, and the apparent patterns of fat deposits. Thus, fat phenotype refers to visible aspects of obesity. Again, the clinical relevance of fat phenotype and putative fat genotype for a given individual is of limited practical importance.

Clearly, there are inherited differences in susceptibility to the risk factors for catabolic maladaptation that leads to obesity. This is quite different from saying that the fat phenotype of a person (visible patterns of fat deposits in the body) is determined predominantly by his fat genotype (hidden genetic coding for fat deposits). To sum this up, when a person wishes to attain and maintain his life span weight, he needs to address all the risk factors of catabolic maladaptation. A genetic susceptibility to catabolic maladaptation (and risk of obesity associated with it) should be looked at simply as that: a susceptibility, an early warning signal.

All of the above can be translated into simple language. When we are overweight or obese, we need not put the blame on our parents. We need to understand that they didn't put obesity in our genes, only a certain susceptibility. Whatever susceptibility they inherited from their parents and passed on to us can be reversed, albeit with a lot of patience and persistence on many occasions.

WHERE DOES OBESITY BEGIN?

My clinical work and research with patients with immune

disorders, chronic fatigue, chemical sensitivity and obesity have led me to the conclusion that the primary site of catabolic maladaptation, and the obesity that it causes, is in the mitochondria. Injury to the mitochondria is primarily inflicted by increased oxidative stress on their structure and function. There is considerable clinical and experimental evidence to support this viewpoint.

Patients with immune disorders, chronic fatigue, chemical sensitivity and obesity almost always show electrophysiologic, biochemical and microscopic profiles indicative of mitochondrial dysfunction. These patients in general show excellent response to nondrug treatment protocols of molecular medicine (environmental medicine, nutritional medicine, medicine of self-regulation and medicine of fitness). With rare exceptions, the most important change my patients observe within 6-12 weeks of initiating treatment with these protocols is higher levels of energy.

The increased level of energy brought about by the treatment protocols of molecular medicine is by far the most telling evidence for improvement in mitochondrial health.

I know many of my physician-colleagues will jump at this statement in anger. They will decry it as subjective and will challenge its validity. I am amazed at how my physician friends are offended by any reference to the subject of energy when treatment protocols used do not include drugs.

When my patients *feel more energetic*, they also show me clear and unequivocal objective laboratory evidence of molecular and immunologic changes. More importantly, my patients begin to reduce the dose of drugs they were taking previously for a variety of diseases previously until they can stop all drugs in most cases.

Now for my scientist-physician colleagues. Many years ago, Peng and co-researchers discovered that mitochondria from the heart muscle which have been deprived of its blood supply are defective in energy (electron) transport and in energy-dependent calcium uptake (J Mol Chem Cardiol 9:897; 1961). This defect in mitochondrial function slows the rate of production of ATP, the principal energy molecule, and, quite literally, causes fatigue. They also made a crucial observation: *The mitochondrial dysfunction —fatigue for the person afflicted by it — can be partially or completely reversed with EDTA chelation therapy.*

Investigations of how mitochondria age in health and disease performed by Gallagher several years earlier had suggested the same, i.e., that EDTA carries the potential for slowing the aging process of mitochondria (Nature 187:162; 1960). EDTA was thought to exert its beneficial effects by chelating (removing) toxic heavy metals as well as excess calcium within the mitochondria. Several subsequent studies clearly showed that mitochondrial health is essential for converting the chemical bond energy of foods into other forms of energy (electrical, osmotic, chemical and mechanical) for the various life processes (*The Mitochondria*, Chapter 13, John Wiley & Sons 1975).

Japanese researchers were the first to report the

increased incidence of DNA deletion in mitochondria of aging cells, sparking intense interest in the role of mitochondria in many other disorders. At present, many of my colleagues at Columbia University are engaged in active mitochondria research looking for a molecular basis of some primary muscle disorders (myopathies) and other muscle disorders such as Parkinson's disease. These and other studies are likely to provide direct experimental evidence for mitochondrial dysfunction in obesity.

The CID State
(A State of Catabolic Insulin Dysregulation)

Sometimes ago I coined the term "catabolic insulin dys-regulation state" to refer to a clinical state of ill-health in which different patterns of symptoms are associated with rapid shifts in blood insulin levels. Insulin dysregulation leads to a host of molecular roller coasters. Some of these molecular highs and lows, such as hypoglycemic troughs and hyperglycemic peaks, are well known to the general public while some others are generally not recognized even by physicians. I generally resist the temptation to coin new terms. There is, however, a real problem for those of us who are focused on the energy and molecular events which initiate illness. The medical jargon has terms only for diseases which it defines based on the cellular and tissue damage *after* it has occurred. The common medical terminology makes no allowance for those who study and treat people *before* the tissues have been damaged. So it is that we, the practitioners of molecular medicine are compelled to coin new terms which express our new *molecular* thinking.

The CID State is responsible for many molecular events which cause symptoms of sudden bouts of weakness, jitteryness, tension, headache, anxiety, mood swings, abdominal discomfort, bloating, flushing, sweating, and difficulties of mood, memory and mentation. The molecular events which trigger these responses include blood sugar roller coasters (rapid hypoglycemic-hyperglycemic shifts), catecholamine surges (rushes of adrenaline and related stress and panic molecules), cholinergic rushes (hormones which hasten to counterbalance excess of adrenaline) and sudden fluctuations in many neurotransmitter levels.

Sugar overload and stress of modern life are important but by no means the main causes of the CID State; oxidized foods and oxidant environmental pollutants, in my view, are equally important.

OBESITY, HEART DISEASE, HYPERTENSION AND DIABETES

The clinical association of these four disorders has been recognized by clinicians and the general public alike for decades. It is common knowledge that many obese people with high blood pressure (hypertension) are able to normalize their blood pressure simply by losing weight. It is also well-known that many obese diabetics can normalize their blood sugar simply by losing weight. The same holds for many people with heart disease. Indeed, weight reduction for such individuals is considered by their physicians as one of the primary treatment strategies (in reality, this is generally a lip service that is followed with a prompt play of the prescription pad).

Only within the last few years have we begun to understand the molecular basis of the association between obesity and hypertension, heart disease, diabetes and many forms of cancer. Several lines of clinical and experimental evidence point to the central role that CID plays in the causation, perpetuation or worsening of these disease states.

What links these four disorders? Dysfunction of insulin and insulin-regulating factors. At first glance, this seems an improbable notion. Hypertension is regarded primarily as a problem of tight arteries. Blood pressure increases as the muscle in the arterial wall tightens, much like the pressure of water contained in a balloon filled with water increases as a child squeezes the balloon. Eventually the balloon bursts. Strokes due to bleeding in the brain that cause motor and sensory deficits (paralysis of limbs and loss of senses) occur in precisely the same way (the blood pressure rises to such a degree that the arterial wall ruptures, spilling blood into the brain substance).

SYNDROME X: A MOLECULAR PUZZLE

Researchers from Stanford University some years ago described the case histories of patients with chest pain and other symptoms of heart disease and abnormal electrocardiograms. They were puzzled by two items: one which they expected but did not find, and the other which they did not expect but did find. The first item was the absence of obstructing plaques in the coronary arteries of the patients. The second item was raised blood levels of insulin. They expressed their surprise by naming this syndrome X.

More studies followed that showed raised levels of insulin

in many people with high blood pressure, raising new questions about the relationship between the two.

Blood insulin levels show abnormalities in almost all people with various types of diabetes and hypoglycemia syndromes. Sometimes these abnormalities are very subtle and are missed by professionals not well-versed in metabolic disorders of insulin. This should not come as a surprise to anyone. After all, everyone knows that insulin is the hormone that regulates blood sugar, and that diabetes and hypoglycemia are problems of sugar regulation.

Now for insulin and obesity. It has been known for many decades that raised levels of insulin increase the rate of turning sugars and proteins into fats. For reasons that are not clear to me, the weight control experts do not see this relationship (or choose to ignore it because it does not serve their dieting strategies).

Catabolic dysregulation of insulin, in essence, is a series of insulin roller coasters. The sharp peaks and deep lows of blood insulin levels are caused by dieting-bingeing cycles, the enormous sugar and salt overload of processed supermarket foods, and by the absence of regular exercise that are essential for insulin regulation. Put in other words, the CID state is but one molecular facet of the catabolic maladaptation I described earlier.

Obesity and Hormones

By far, the most common hormonal abnormality associated with catabolic maladaptation in obesity is the catabolic insulin dysregulation that I discussed at some length in the preceding paragraphs.

The incidence of endocrine diseases as causes of obesity in the general public, as defined in classical medical literature, is extremely low. When endocrine glandular lesions do occur, the total clinical picture often contains clear clues to their existence. Advances in laboratory technologies have made the accurate diagnosis of such disorders a simple matter. Unless such clues exist, extensive and expensive laboratory tests for obese people are neither necessary nor useful. It is a far superior strategy to systematically search for and address all the risk factors of catabolic maladaptation. This is essential even on those few occasions when endocrine lesions do exist. In the catabolic maladaptive state, however, I frequently observe clinical and laboratory evidence of significant dysfunction of three endocrine glands: the thyroid gland (cold hands and feet and low energy), the pancreas (troublesome hypoglycemia-hyperglycemia shifts), and the adrenal gland (the chronic stress state).

I include the following survey of hormonal imbalances that are observed in obese persons as general information for the reader. In general, they occur as the *consequences* and not the causes of obesity.

The Thyroid Gland

Insufficient amounts of thyroxine (hypothyroidism) cause weight gain and lead to serious obesity if not corrected. From a practical standpoint, however, this is not a difficult problem to resolve. Hypothyroidism is an easy disorder to diagnose clinically and with some laboratory tests. The commonly used T3, T4, T7 and TSH tests sometimes fail to detect early evolving cases of hypothyroidism. The newer sensitive fluorescent antibody tests for antithyroid antibodies are very useful in the diagnosis of such subtle cases.

The Pituitary Gland and Growth Hormone

Output of growth hormone by the pituitary gland is decreased in obesity. This occurs both under resting conditions as well as when the pituitary gland is stimulated by growth hormone-releasing hormone (GHRH) of the hypothalamus. Likewise, the increase in the blood levels of growth hormone that is normally seen during sleep, fasting, and exercise, and with high-protein meals is decreased in obesity.

The Pituitary-Ovary Axis

The pituitary-ovary axis in women frequently shows signs of imbalance in obese women. The incidence of menstrual irregularities, early menarche (menstruation), delayed menopause, and hirsutism (excessive hair on the face and other parts of the body) is higher in obese women than in women with normal weights. Obese women have a higher incidence of cancer of the uterus.

What is the molecular basis of these hormonal abnormalities? In post-menopausal women, almost all estrogen and related female hormones are produced from testosterone and related male hormones. The conversion of male hormones to female hormones occurs mostly in fat cells and connective tissue cells that hold the fat cells together. The increased number and size of fat cells in obesity increase the rate of this turnover, and lead to various consequences of hormonal imbalance. Similar events occur in premenopausal women, though to a lesser degree.

The Pituitary-Testis Axis

The pituitary-testis axis is abnormal in obesity. Obese persons often have oligospermia (low sperm count) and aspermia (absence of sperms in semen). Obese men have lower levels of testosterone and frequently show raised levels of estrogen. Indeed, there is some indication that a low estrogen level is one of the risk factors for coronary artery disease for such individuals.

The Hypothalamus-Pituitary-Adrenal Axis

The hypothalamus-pituitary-adrenal axis in both males and females appears not to show gross abnormalities detectable with current laboratory methods. In health, the hypothalamus in the brain regulates pituitary activity by releasing a hormone called corticotrophin-releasing hormone. The pituitary gland, in turn, regulates the activity of the adrenal gland by releasing a hormone called corticotrophin (ACTH). The blood levels of the adrenal hormone called cortisol provide the necessary negative feedback to the hypothalamus. Even though these relationships appear to be intact in obesity, subtle abnormalities do occur that add to the problems of energy and general well-being.

The Parathyroid Gland

Recent studies have uncovered an unexpected finding in the parathyroid function in obesity. The blood levels of the parathyroid gland hormone called parahormone are raised. Urinary cyclic AMP (a marker for parathyroid activity) is also increased in obesity. Obese people often have low blood levels of vitamin D and show evidence of osteoporosis. It seems probable that the parathyroid gland overacts (usually without success) to correct these disorders.

Endorphin, Vasopressin and Norepinephrine

Some other changes in tissues levels of certain hormones

and neurotransmitters in obesity have been reported. The role that changes play in the cause of obesity is not clear at this time. These include the following: 1) beta-endorphin that exerts significant effects on feeding behavior; 2) vasopressin, a hormone that controls water balance; and 3) norepinephrine that is an important stress and panic molecule (a close cousin molecule to adrenaline).

The most important point to be made in this discussion of hormonal imbalances in obesity is that they are caused by obesity. They do not cause obesity. Almost all of these changes can be reversed with time when the life span weight is attained and maintained. Rarely do tumors or other lesions of the endocrine glands cause obesity, and these are generally easy to diagnose.

Obesity Is But One Facet of the Catabolic Maladaptation

In closing this section, I will summarize the biochemical changes involved with a few brief comments about the true nature of the problem of obesity.

Obesity is but one sign of a catabolic disorder (which I call catabolic maladaptation in this volume). In this disorder, the ability of muscles to burn fat is diminished, and fat accumulates in the body. There are four principal reasons for this:

First,

the fat cells that store fat and the muscle fibers that burn fat become toxic with oxidized and toxic fats. Toxic fat cells become sluggish and bloated. Some fats like trans fatty acids found in margarine cannot be metabolized by human enzymes.

Second,

muscle mass is reduced. Since fat breakdown primarily occurs in muscles, reduced muscle mass cannot cope with increasing demands for burning fat. Thus, more fat accumulates in tissues.

Third,

sluggish muscles struggle with sluggish enzymes. Active muscles carry active enzymes. Enzymes are essential for urning fat. Some of these muscle enzymes are poisoned by toxic fats and others by toxic metals and environmental pollutants.

Fourth,

many hormones in the body function to clear fat from the fat cells. Fat accumulates in fat cells when these hormones are weakened or inactivated by toxic heavy metals, environmental pollutants, pesticides, certain viruses and other agents. Malnutrition, stress and panic, pain disorders and immune dysfunctions are other factors leading to hormonal insufficiency. Excess and the imbalance of insulin caused by sugar overload cause fat to accumulate in fat cells. The same holds for stress and panic molecules such as adrenaline and its cousin molecules, lactic acid.

SOME COMMONLY ASKED QUESTIONS

I am frequently asked questions about obesity. Below some of those questions followed by brief answers.

Question:

What is the true nature of obesity?

Answer:

Obesity is one of the symptoms of *catabolic maladaptation.*

Question:

What is catabolic maladaptation?

Answer:

Catabolic maladaptation is a disorder of metabolism in which the fat cells in the body become toxic with fats. The muscle fibers atrophy. Fat-burning enzymes are poisoned by toxic foods, environmental pollutants and pernicious molecules produced by the stress of an accelerated lifestyle. These molecular events cause cellular fatigue. Fatigue leads to inactivity, which in turn feeds these molecular loops. The nature, causes, progression and strategies of reversal of this maladaptation are discussed in the chapter, The Catabolic Maladaptation.

Question:

What are toxic fats?

Answer:

Toxic fats are oxidized and injured fats that fat cells cannot catabolize. These fats include trans fatty acids, toxic cyclic fats and peroxides of fatty acids. All hydrogenated oils, margarines, shortenings and fats processed with industrial solvents contain toxic fats.

Question:

Do micronutrients such as vitamins and minerals play any role in the causation and maintenance of obesity?

Answer:

Yes. These essential nutrients do play important roles in the causation and maintenance of obesity. However, the critical point is this: In the general population, micronutrients play *secondary* roles. Toxic fats, sugar overload and down-regulation of fat-burning enzymes play the *primary* roles.

Question:

How can we control obesity?

Answer:

By reversing catabolic maladaptation with life span foods, environmental controls, limbic exercise and self-regulation.

Question:

How do the popular concepts of dieting experts relating to neuropsychology, neurophysiology, and neurobiology for weight loss relate to the concept of catabolic maladaptation?

Answer:

These concepts have some positive aspects as well as some misleading aspects.

The positive aspects are that they help us to look at obesity in a larger perspective. We can understand the roles played by the hypothalamus and the limbic areas in the nervous system, neurotransmitters in the brain and other tissues, and the anxiety, stress and panic molecules.

What is misleading about these concepts is that they look to the mind for answers to the problems of the fat cells bloated with oxidized, denatured fats, emaciated muscle fibers, the energy-generating and energy-expending enzyme systems.

DIAGNOSIS OF OBESITY

How can obesity be clinically diagnosed? The weight control experts love to debate this issue. They use complicated formulas that only they can understand.

I have a simple working (and clinically useful) definition for obesity. *Obesity is the presence of any fat which a person does not need to live his life span with energy, vigor and perfect health.* By this definition, a person should aim to be as lean, firm and robust as he can be. In that state, he is not obese. Being simply thin is not enough. Undernourished and emaciated children, adult alcoholics, anorectics and bulimic are thin but listless and tired individuals. Simple thinness is not what we are after. It is thinness with other essentials for living a full life span that is the key.

There are several methods of determining body fat content. Dieting experts love to extol the virtues of their favorite methodology as they vehemently find faults with those used by their opponents.

What is lost in all this unnecessary controversy is the essence of the matter: Unnecessary fat is an unnecessary biologic burden on the body. Oxidized, denatured fats clog the molecular wheels of health. But the truth stated in such a simple, unpretentious way is not acceptable to the experts. There is no room for debate here. Experts need complex numerical values so that they can develop complicated formulas and equations for elegant bits of computing. Armed with such "data," they are now ready to dismiss anyone wishing to talk common sense as simpleminded, or worse, feebleminded.

My suggested guidelines for life span weights for women and men are given in tables included in the chapter, Life Span Weight. This information is intended only as a *guideline*. In the life span perspective defined here, the life span weight for a given person must be determined by him or her alone, through limbic listening to tissues for energy, vigor and health. The values included in the tables, laboratory assessment of total body fat and professional advice are all very valuable, but none of them is a substitute for limbic listening to catabolic signals from within.

MEASUREMENT OF LEAN BODY WEIGHT AND TOTAL BODY WEIGHT

Accurate measurements of lean body mass and total body fat are very valuable during the initial evaluation and for monitoring the progress in a weight control program with focus on life span issues.

The best and most practical method for determining total

body fat and lean body mass is with bioelectric impedance technology. For general interest, I also include the following brief comments about other commonly used methodologies for the determination of total body fat and lean body weight.

Anthropometric Measurements

This method of determining the existence and degree of obesity is based on measurements of height and weight. A simple formula used by many insurance companies calculates the relative weight by dividing the person's weight by a standard weight value based upon his height. The standard weights used for this approach are generally those published by the Metropolitan Life Insurance Company. The Metropolitan standard weights are "based on the weight associated with the lowest mortality at any given height." This method has been used in many studies including the Framingham studies. Nevertheless, several objections to this method have been raised over the years. Clearly this approach does not use one standard for all patients.

A second approach is to calculate the weight-height index (WHI). The WHI is calculated by dividing the weight with some power of height, the power to be used being selected for a population to give the maximum correlation with body fat and the minimum correlation with body height. A commonly used formula is kg per m^2 (kilogram per meter).

Underwater Weighing Method

According to the principle of Archimedes (the Greek mathematician), the volume of a body can be calculated from the difference between its weight in air and its weight in water. This method requires that the subject be totally immersed in water for the determination of body fat weight — not a very practical approach in clinical medicine.

Skin Fold Methods

For many years, the methods based on skin fold thickness measurements were used in obesity clinics. These methods have the advantage in that no equipment is necessary except for special calipers. Measurements taken with calipers have to be entered into some formulas to obtain usable data. From a practical standpoint, these older methods are not as desirable as the newer methods based on bioelectric impedance.

Radioisotope Methods

Radioisotopic methods are accurate methods for use in research but are too cumbersome to be of much practical use in clinical medicine. Of course these methods require giving the subject a dose of radioactive material which is neither desirable nor practical for clinical programs for better health through weight loss.

Impedance Technology

Lean body mass and total body fat can be measured with electronic equipment. The noninvasive procedure causes no pain or discomfort. In this test the results obtained with impedance electronic technology for lean body mass, fat body mass and body water weight are entered into a computer. The data for the individual's body weight, body height and the aerobic exercise status are also fed into the computer. A complete analysis so performed is used as one of the bases for designing a nutrition and an exercise protocol for an individual.

Bioelectrical impedance technology represents one of the most important recent advances in preventive medicine. For the first time it is now possible to perform a complete analysis of lean body weight, body fat weight and body water weight by an efficient, cost-effective and noninvasive technology. Impedance refers to the resistance that tissues offer to the passage of an electrical impulse. Of the various body tissues, impedance is greatest in fatty tissues. The tissues included in the lean body weight (such as muscles and bones) have a high content of water and minerals, and hence allow the passage of electrical impulses with much less resistance. This physical phenomenon is the basis for the determination of the body composition with an impedance analyzer system that I use in my clinical work. The results obtained with this technology have shown to be more accurate and reproducible than conventional time-consuming and expensive methodologies in several research centers in the country.

Body Composition Analysis

In this analysis, information obtained by the electrical impedance analyzer is fed to the computer along with data about the patient's age, weight, height, level of general physical activity and the results of aerobic exercise evaluation. A comprehensive computer analysis is then performed to obtain the following information:

1. Accurate measurement of lean body mass.
2. Accurate measurement of body fat mass.
3. Accurate measurement of total body water.
4. Accurate measurement of lean to fat mass ratio for ideal lean to fat ratio for the individual.
5. Comparison of the ideal lean to fat ratio of the individual with the normal ranges observed in different patient populations.
6. Estimation of basal metabolism rate.
7. Aerobic evaluation.
8. Specific recommendations for calorie consumption.
9. Specific recommendations for exercise.
10. Personalized weight loss chart based on all the above findings.

Precautions for Lean Mass Analysis

1. Alcoholic beverages should not be taken in the 24-hour period before the test.

2. Physical exercise should not be done in the 12-hour period before the test

3. Meals should not be eaten in the 4-hour period before the test.

4. Water and other fluids should be taken as normally for a period of 24 hours before the test. It is important to avoid dehydration as well as overhydration

OPTIMAL LEAN BODY MASS

To live fit is to be fit, fit in mind and fit in spirit. And the road to wellness of the mind and spirit starts with fitness of body. This is an ancient truism and it is as true today as it was in ancient times, although there are now some differences.

The ancients did not breathe our polluted air, drink our contaminated water and eat our depleted foods. Their biology was not challenged each day by aging-oxidant molecules the way ours is.

The best approach to fitness of body is by achieving and maintaining life span weight with optimal ratios between lean body weight, body fat weight and body water weight. In most instances, increase in body weight results from an increase in body fat predominantly. By contrast, in most cases weight loss includes the loss of body fat as well as lean body weight. Thus, it is essential to analyze these body weight compartments carefully in all programs designed to lose or gain total body weight.

LEAN BODY WEIGHT

Lean body weight includes muscles, bones, tendons, connective tissue and various body organs excluding the fat content of these tissues. In most individuals, water represents 71% to 75% of lean body weight. In the past, lean body weight could be measured indirectly by measuring the total body weight and estimating the body fat.

BODY FAT

Some body organs such as breasts and tissues under the skin are almost exclusively composed of fatty tissues. In addition, fat is found in variable amounts in most organs of the body such as the heart, muscles, bones and other tissues. In general, fatty tissues in all such locations are increased in obese individuals and decreased in thin persons. Fourteen percent to 22% of the fatty tissue in the body is composed of water.

TOTAL BODY WATER

Measurement of total body water is an essential step in any body composition analysis. The water content of various tissues differs widely. As indicated previously, 71% to 75% of lean body weight is composed of water while water content of fatty tissues ranges from 14% to 22%.

The measurement of total body water is done by using a very complex isotope dilution analysis. These analyses require very expensive equipment and are very cumbersome and time-consuming.

CHANGES IN LEAN BODY WEIGHT AND ENERGY EXPENDITURE DURING WEIGHT LOSS

Life span weight is regulated by several functional aspects of the myocyte and the adipocyte discussed earlier in this section. The two principal elements are an ample supply of life span foods and adequate limbic lipolytic activity.

Extensive research has shown that attempts to lose

weight by caloric restriction result in loss of body lean mass as well as body fat mass. Several factors determine how much weight loss will result from the loss of body fat and how much from body lean mass. Further, the amount of body fat loss and body lean mass loss are different in the initial and late phases of a weight loss program.

Another important concept in this context is the loss of *labile proteins*. Labile proteins are nonstructural proteins that consume energy and are important for essential biologic functions in the heart, liver, intestine, skin and other organs. Simple restriction of calories as is done in the popular dieting programs results in adaptive hormonal responses that reduce the rate of protein synthesis.

RESTING ENERGY EXPENDITURE

The term resting energy expenditure (REE) refers to the amount of energy spent by the body to maintain essential life functions in a state of rest. Dieting (caloric restriction in weight loss programs) results in a reduction of resting energy expenditure in both lean and overweight individuals.

Overweight individuals who participate in various popular diet programs usually lose some weight during the initial period. Within some weeks, these people find that the early success in weight reduction is not maintained. This results from a decrease in the REE rate. Dieting also reduces REE in lean individuals. With continued dieting, the rate of protein loss is reduced somewhat and that of fat loss is maintained. Notwithstanding, considerable loss of lean body tissue continues to occur during prolonged dieting in all people.

MONITORING BODY LEAN MASS

It should be evident from the preceding comments how important continuous monitoring of body lean mass is in optimum weight management and weight reduction protocols. Clearly, the objectives are to maintain optimal lean body mass for essential life functions as unwanted pounds in body fat are shed. Following are four important issues:

1. Caloric restriction to lose body fat mass.
2. Nutritional strategy to maintain optimal body lean mass.
3. Ample supply of all essential micronutrients.
4. An exercise program designed to up-regulate catabolic enzymes and preserve lean body mass.

The newer electroconductance technology has made precise monitoring of lean body mass both practical and cost-effective. It has replaced the cumbersome, time-consuming and expensive methodologies of past years.

In closing this chapter, I return to the butterfly. The problem of obesity can be solved only through a true understanding of the nature of this problem. As Choua says so often, our mitochondria do not recognize our silly notions of fad diets. Our lipase enzymes have not yet discovered our invention of the refrigerator or our food stamp programs. Our ATP molecules do not have much use for the frozen packed foods that merchants of the dieting industry foist on us with sizzling commercials of women in bikinis running on beaches. Our cell membranes are defenseless against assault by toxic fats in our French fries and greasy hamburgers.

"Our study confirms that childhood obesity is a major problem," she says. "Fifty percent more children today are overweight than were ten years ago."

Wendy Wolfe
Cornell Alumni News March 1992, page 12

Before our children can fly up and out, they first have to see the skylight of oxidized, denatured and toxic fats thrown before them by our food industry. How can our children learn this when our adults don't? How can our adults know this when the high priests of medicine at the American Heart Association don't?

What we need is not a low-fat diet but a no-oxidized, no-denatured fat diet. As I write this, my eyes fall upon the brochure *Recipes for Low-Fat, Low-Cholesterol Meals* published by American Heart Association. It is full of recipes that use margarine. Margarine has up to 35% of its fats as trans fatty acids that our body cannot use. What we do by eating margarine is to give our cells a coat of *plastic fats* and, quite literally, suffocate them. It is well-known that trans fatty acids raise LDL cholesterol and lower HDL (*N Eng J Med* 323:439; 1990), but this, of course, does not seem to be of any concern to the folks at the American Heart Association.

We physicians have our own skylights.

Chapter 5

Stress,
Obesity And the
Language of Silence

Some obesity experts believe obesity is repressed anger turned into fat globules. They think childhood anguish metamorphoses into fatty acids that accumulate in fat cells as triglycerides. Parental neglect materializes into fatty tissue in children. When we grow up, childhood memories condense into cellulite in thighs and hips. Interesting points of view!

Then there are others who believe the human organism is nothing but diffuse consciousness that sometimes takes form as limbs attached to a torso with a head poised above them on a pedestal of neck. The problem begins when this consciousness is ignored. A smitten consciousness, the disciples of this *expanded* view of cosmic existence assert, takes its revenge, and layers the tissues with chunks of fat. These layers of fat cannot be simply peeled off with simplistic notions of exercise and healthful food. What is required is an extended, a very extended cosmic reach for the diffused consciousness. The errant cosmic consciousness must be captured, brought down to earth, and be persuaded to reshape us into desired lithesome bodies. Fascinating stuff!

Many of my patients suffer from severe anxiety states, panic attacks and depression. Their pain is unremitting. They know something about *human suffering*. In caring for them I have made some observations. Many of them gain some weight when their troubles become deep and most lose some weight initially as their clinical state improves. Then their weight stabilizes. My basic observation has been this: *Those who started out with up-regulated enzymes, by and large, keep their enzymes up-regulated and gained little weight even when their suffering becomes intense and unrelenting. Those who started with down-regulated enzymes often became obese.*

"My greatest failure was in believing that the weight issue was just about weight. It's not. It's about not handling stress properly. It's about sexual abuse. It's about all the things that cause other people to become alcoholics and drug addicts....... If you lose weight on a diet, sooner or later you'll gain it back...... I used to brag,"I don't ever get stress." I'd ask,"What is stress? What does it feel like?" The reason I didn't feel stressed is that I ate my way through it."

Oprah Winfrey in "The Pain of Regain"
Quoted in *People* magazine. Jan. 14, 1991

The butterfly yearns to fly up and out. The skylight of down-regulated enzymes doesn't let her. She cannot fly through the glass. She needs to fly down and in before you she can fly up and out of the skylight frame. This she cannot see. Catabolic maladaptation spreads a cruel net of molecular deception before her.

Ms. Winfrey evidently is not a student of biology. Catabolic maladaptation is a severe biologic handicap. Dieting is exactly the wrong thing to do. Dieting cannot work, and it didn't for her.

What is in common with obesity, malaria, tumors of the parathyroid gland, steroid psychosis, alcoholism and cocaine addiction? What is in common between obesity and the Chemical Sensitivity Syndrome?

Malaria causes spikes of high fever, chills, vomiting and muscle pains. What could bring upon a poor soul such affliction, common folks wondered in medieval times? Only evil spirits could unleash such misery, they reasoned. Malaria became a disease of evil spirits.

How were tumors of the parathyroid gland first recognized? This is a forgotten subject now. The parathyroid glands are four pea-sized glands which lie covered by the thyroid gland in the neck. Some persons with tumors of the parathyroid glands, which usually remain small and invisible, were incarcerated in asylums because they were regarded insane by the medical "authorities" of their time. Some parathyroid tumors became very large and visible. A surgeon became interested in them and removed some of them. To his great surprise, some of these patients made a complete recovery from their mental illness. The medical profession learned something important: There can be an *organic* cause of mental illness.

Psychosis is sometimes caused by steroids. How was this discovered? Some people who were prescribed steroids became psychotic. The psychiatrists *firmly* established their diagnoses of specific psychiatric disorders, and put these patients on their "drugs of choice" for specific types of mental illness. When steroids were discontinued, their psychiatric illness disappeared. A triumph of synthetic chemistry! I can almost hear some psychiatrist or chemist croon with victory. When enough of these victories had been celebrated, someone noticed the relationship between discontinuance of steroids and cures of psychosis. We learned something else: Chemicals can cause for mental illness.

Alcoholics were sinners. The righteous had their days of glory. That, of course, was before advances in neurotransmitter chemistry unravelled the chemical mystery of alcoholism. We learned a new lesson: Moral problems can have a molecular basis. Cocaine addicts were criminal. Criminologists congratulated themselves for their great insights into criminal minds. Advances in neuroreceptor chemistry spoiled all that. We learned crime can be chemically provoked.

I return to my question. What is in common with obesity, malaria, parathyroid tumors, alcoholism and cocaine addiction? The answer: Silly notions of health and disease. Absence of knowledge of our biology gives people freedom to imagine, and the imagination of people in the *mind business* are often very fertile. Fortunately, science has a way of dispensing with foolish notions about health and diseases.

What does obesity have in common with the multiple chemical sensitivity syndrome? This syndrome is still regarded by many medical "authorities" as obsessional psychopathology. Big words! Slender intellects! Ignorance of biology. Funny notions of the causes of human suffering. What I find incredible about the multiple chemical sensitivity syndrome is that so many of our distinguished professors from some of our most prestigious universities dismiss the concept of chemical sensitivity as a problem of the mind. They insult the physicians (clinical ecologists) who try to relate a patient's suffering to chemicals in his environments. The professors call clinical ecologists cultists. I wonder what these professors will say when, in some years, the scientific proof for molecular injury inflicted by chemicals in minute quantities will be established? Both are widely misunderstood subjects. Both are mislabelled as problems of the mind.

Obesity is also regarded by many "authorities" as a problem of the mind. Many professionals believe that the problem of obesity can be solved by keeping the mouth shut for dieting or, taking a contrary viewpoint, by opening it to spill out their guts and let out the hidden anger and hostility.

Many medical specialties profit from their own incompetence. Bariatrics, the specialty which deals with obesity, tops this list in my view. Usually they start off with what they consider are comprehensive and integrated physical, mental and spiritual approaches to the problem of obesity. They have elaborate schemes for venting reservoirs of anger and hostility, and they carry elegant diet pills and potions to dispense to their patients. When the patient is exhausted (in more than one way), they invoke the stress theory and deftly put the blame on the patient. Obesity, they pronounce, is a problem of the mind, and hence a responsibility of the patient.

Obesity is a catabolic maladaptation caused by definable molecular and energy events. Obesity is no more *caused* by stress or anxiety than is allergy caused by these factors. It is true that stress, anxiety, panic, sexual abuse, substance abuse and other related disorders can compound the problem of obesity, just as these factors increase the intensity of allergy symptoms. But there must be no mistake about the true nature of obesity and allergy. Obesity is a catabolic maladaptation, a failure of mitochondrial energy enzymes, just as allergy is a genetic programming to react to molecules in our environment.

Are there more nervous fat people than there are nervous thin people? Is stress a greater problem for obese people than it is for the thin? Are there more fat sexually abused people than there are thin sexually abused people?

Ask a thin person. Stressful situations usually depress his hunger; calamities make him anorectic. Then ask a fat person. Stress makes him overeat. Why does a thin person choose to starve himself when he is stressed? Why does a fat person binge when he is stressed? The answers to these questions, it seems to me, have something to do with the state of their enzymes. Up-regulated enzymes stay up-regulated even during periods of less eating. Down-regulated enzymes seem not to be able to do so. The enthusiasts of the stress theory of obesity are unburdened by any knowledge of human biology and enzyme energy dynamics.

STRESS MOLECULES
ARE POWERFUL OXIDANT MOLECULES

The issue of stress in modern life is very real. In my experience, mind-over-body methods for dissipating stress generally do not give good results. Autoregulation based on demonstrable electrophysiologic energy changes in the body (a body-over-mind strategy) and similar time-honored methods of self-regulation, offer superior clinical results.

Life in our time is an unending sequence of stresses. Before we can recover from one stressor, we are confronted with another. What we commonly call stress is a highly complex mosaic of interrelated molecular events. The well known adrenaline molecules, and its less known cousin molecules, catecholamines, are powerful oxidant molecules. These molecules, and other potent oxyradicals produced by them, poke holes in cell membranes. It matters little whether these molecular events are triggered by anger, hostility, anxiety, panic or stress. What is inside the cell hemorrhages out; what is outside floods the cell innards. Cellular enzymes are injured, poisoned and paralyzed. This is the beginning of the catabolic maladaptation. Stress, seen in this light, is of great relevance to the true cause of obesity, catabolic maladaptation.

We seldom realize that this process of oxidative molecular injury, which causes catabolic maladaptation, is identical to that caused by toxic foods, allergy, chemical sensitivity, viral infections, chronic fatigue and degenerative disorders. All these states lead to the production of potent oxyradicals which poke holes in the cell membranes and paralyze mitochondrial energy enzymes.

Equally important is the issue of what to do about stress in reversing the catabolic maladaptation. Excessive build-up of stress molecules must be prevented with all relevant strategies. This is as necessary for obese people as it is for thin persons. The essential problem of obesity is not that people do not realize the absolute need for exercise or for proper eating. The essential problem is that they are put on diets that do not work, and are told to exercise in ways that are unsuitable for them. I discuss the subjects of food choices and exercise later in this volume. I describe the methods of autoregulation that I find clinically most useful in my books *The Cortical Monkey and Healing* and *Directed Pulses*. I include here some excerpts from the former to express my personal observations on this subject.

STRESS: A MAJOR MALADY OF OUR TIME

Self-regulation cannot be a purely intellectual pursuit; healing cannot be forced upon our tissues when we are in the cortical state. It happens when we listen to them in the limbic state.

The first core idea of autoregulation requires that we fully understand the nature of the disease; the second, that we begin to explore our biology, learn to regulate our body organs, and finally reverse our diseases. Some people balk at the term "self-healing." This is unnecessary semantic hassling. Healing is a natural phenomenon. Tissues have an innate capacity for healing. We physicians are not healers. We only use our knowledge of healing arts to remove impediments in the way of tissue healing.

Autoregulation requires a shift from the usual mind-set of wanting control over our circumstances, the cortical mode, to one of insight and harmony with our biology, the limbic mode. The cortical mode is the thinking mode. The *limbic mode* is the feeling (and healing) mode. The difference between these two modes is very real and critical to success in self-healing.

In our autoregulation laboratory, I regularly observe, predictably and reproducibly, how the manner by which a person attends to his own thoughts and feelings determines the state of his biology. He stresses his biology when he enters the cortical mode. He calms and rests his biology when he settles into the limbic mode. We have a choice:

We can perpetuate a chronic illness by speaking about it, forever analyzing it, and suppressing its symptoms with drugs.

Or

We can heal an illness by listening to our biology, responding to it, and regulating it.

Western culture, in some ways, can be seen as a culture of confession. We often believe that to speak is to heal. To name a disease is to understand it. To classify a disease is to conquer it. To use drugs for a disease is to cure it. This model served us well when we fought against polio, smallpox and other infectious diseases. But is it applicable to the vast majority of diseases we fight today? Is the prevailing practice of drug medicine relevant to illnesses caused by problems of nutrition, stress, environmental pollutants, and fitness? These are important questions for people in and out of healing arts.

Self-regulation offers a person an alternative. It offers a choice between speaking and drugging tissues for control of a disease and listening and responding for insights into the inner workings of tissues and their healing processes.

PSYCHOSOMATIC AND SOMATOPSYCHIC MODELS OF DISEASES ARE ARTIFACTS OF OUR THINKING.

Diseases are burdens on our biology. Psyche (mind) and soma (body) are inseparable parts of our biology. This debate between psychosomatic and somatopsychic models of disease is futile. It generates much heat but creates no light. As we become more enlightened in our biologic perspectives, I believe, this debate will die out.

Advances in behavioral biology and experimental psychology are putting these two disciplines on a collision course. Neuroanatomists are mapping out the human brain by defining the neurotransmitter's pathways. They are creating what Bartley Hoebel of Princeton University calls "a new psychological taxonomy based on chemical neuroanatomy." We are witnessing the dawn of a new science: *the science of oneness of the body and mind.*

Stress is an integral part of our biology. Stress can trigger, mimic, or exaggerate almost all disease processes. In biology, the stress response is an essential element of an organism's physiology. We cannot live without this response any more than we can live without a heart beating in our chest, or a brain creating impulses in our skulls. The stress response is composed of an interrelated series of electromagnetic and physicochemical events. These events throw our whole biology into a more strained state. Our pain becomes more acute, our suffering more intense. Success in autoregulation requires that we begin with success in stress control.

Focus on the biologic aspects of stress, and not the analysis of its cause, is a superior strategy when we are under stress.

Knowledge of the cause of stress is essential for the prevention of stress. But this knowledge, by itself, cannot dissipate stress for us. Focus on the biologic consequences of the stress response (the condition of the heart, brain and other body functions) gives far superior clinical benefits than any emphasis on the analysis of its cause. Specifically, in the methods of autoregulation, we focus on the state of various body organs to obtain a more consistent and predictable control of stress.

The problem for people is not the absence of desire to control stress, it is not knowing *how* to do it. Telling a patient under stress to relax is akin to telling a patient with a migraine attack to dissolve his headache without a drug. If he could do so, he would not be suffering the way he is. For most patients in the throes of chronic illness and unremitting stress, the word "relax" does not carry any images for control of the biologic stress reactions.

By common life experience, we know what it means to be "relaxed", a state of physical and mental calm. By common experience, we also know that this alone does not help us in controlling stress.

One essential aspect of stress which is often not fully recognized is that all the adverse effects of the stress response do not wear off soon after the stressor is removed. Indeed, in the diseases initiated, perpetuated, and worsened by stress, the intermediate and long-term effects of stress are much more important than the immediate effects.

The intermediate and long-term effects of the stress response are the root causes of many of the diseases of our time, including the catabolic maladaptation. The stress response puts our whole biology in high gear, a state of *biologic burnout*. What we call stress in common language is a highly complex and delicately balanced series of electromagnetic and biochemical events. It causes anxiety, rapid heart rate, heart palpitations, sweating, abdominal cramps, diarrhea, muscle spasms, high blood pressure, spastic colitis, and eventually leads to chronic fatigue syndrome, stomach ulcers, heart disease and a host of other disorders.

In clinical medicine, we can address the problem of how to control stress either by *clever* thinking or by a considered strategy of *absence of thinking*. In my own clinical work with autoregulation, I find the latter approach much more effective than the former. Specifically, I teach my patients how to bring about the desired electrophysiological changes to dissipate the stress molecules with a *biologic-intuitive* approach. I teach them simple methods for observing and exploring their biology. I use the term "Biologic Profile" for a composite picture which graphically demonstrates to the patient the structure and function of his various body tissues.

These biologic profiles are true-to-life, precise and accurate images of electromagnetic, molecular, and microscopic events which occur in a patient's biology in health and disease. Our technology allows us to look at living cells, tissues, and organs. In my own clinical work I focus on those methods where a person can see what is abnormal, respond to it, and then see for himself the effects of his efforts. Other technologies such as pictures of ovaries taken with a laparoscope (an instrument used to examine the inside of the belly) or snapshots of a stomach ulcer taken with a gastroscope are also very useful even though these are not suitable for seeing immediate responses to the methods of self-regulation.

A biologic profile of a patient may consist of moving integrated graphs showing the activity of various body organs. We describe for our patients the significance of each of the components in these profiles. We ask our patients to observe their own profiles. We explain to them the meaning of each of the elements of these graphs. Next, we teach them simple methods for effecting a change in the functions of these organs. This is followed by instruction in the specific methods for treating specific diseases. In essence, this is what we mean by observation and exploration of our biology.

The biologic profile for a patient may be limited and confined to two or three body organs, or it may be comprehensive and integrate the details of several organs simultaneously on a single computer screen. Specifically, biologic profiles can be designed to include the heart rate and rhythm, patterns of circulation, activity in different parts of the brain, electrical charges in the muscles, and levels of energy (galvanic or conductance) in skin responses. The following illustration is an example of a biologic profile for a patient with severe stress.

The biologic profile shown below graphically demonstrates the difference between an even, restorative state of some tissues in a limbic mode and a stressful condition of same tissues in a cortical mode. The graph lines from top to bottom indicate the functional state of muscles (2 lines representing two electrodes on muscles of an arm), heart, arteries and skin conductance energy. The first phase of the graph shows a period when the person was doing autoregulation. Both muscle lines show a gradual slope downward that reflects a progressive decrease in wasteful tension in the muscles. The line in the middle demonstrates a regular rhythm of the heart with gentle wave-like pattern. The fourth line from above shows an open state of the arteries in the finger that carries the plathysmograph sensor. This line also shows a gentle rhythmic wave-like activity in the arterial walls. The straight line at the bottom shows an even state of electrodermal conductance energy. Viewed as a group of organ, this biologic profile represents a steady state of biology — a restorative state of organ function that is free of any cortical overdrive.

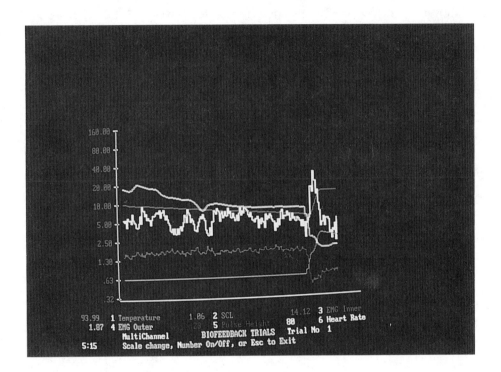

The abrupt swings in the graph lines near the end of the profile occurred as the subject in this study stopped autoregulation and tried to see how his profile looked and understand what the various graphs meant. The arterial line (second from below) shows a nosedive representing sudden constriction of arteries caused by cortical constrictive impulses from the vasomotor center in the brain, a classical example of the workings of the cortical monkey. Next, the heart is forced to respond to sudden tightening of the arteries. It, quite literally, heaves under stress as it strains to force blood through tightened arteries. This is how hypertension (high blood pressure) begins. The changes in the arterial and heart lines are rapidly accompanied by equally abrupt changes in the muscle and skin graphs. An even, steady-state, restorative, limbic state of biology is switched to a turbulent, stressful, disease-causing cortical state.

The message given by this biologic profile to its owner, the patient wired to the computer screen with electronic sensors, is simple, loud, and clear. The way he attends to his own cortical (intellectual) thoughts or listens to (and responds) to his tissues determines the state of his biology. In matters of body tissues and cells under the skin, the mind often deceives; the tissues and cells never learned how to lie.

He has a choice:

He can choose the cortical mode, keep his biology in turbulence, perpetuate his state of dis-ease and become ill.

Or

He can choose the limbic mode, keep his biology at an even pace, self-regulate and heal.

OBESITY AMONG TRIBAL PEOPLE

There are almost no obese people in tribal Africa and tribal Asia.

There were almost no obese people among the American Indians and Alaskan Eskimos. Now obesity is pervasive among both American ethnic groups. On closer examination, the risk factors for catabolic maladaptation were few or nonexistent in American Indians and Eskimos until they were introduced to a "modern, enriched diet." Some enrichment! Enriched in oxidized and denatured fats, enriched in oxidized and denatured proteins, enriched in oxidized and devitalized vitamins, enriched in heavy metal immunotoxicants, overloaded with sugars and laced with salt. Enriched in molecules that poison mitochondrial enzymes. Enriched in injured foods that injure cells. Enriched in materials that rob people of fluidity of motion and spontaneity in action. Enriched in alcohol and enriched in mind-altering drugs. Devastated by our "enriched" foods, disabled by incapacitating fatigue, dazed with alcohol, and mauled by obesity, these American Indians and Alaskan Eskimos are now ready (albeit unwilling) for our analytic couches. We study them as sociologic phenomena. We make eloquent pronouncements about "cross-cultural dynamics", and invoke elegant models of obesity caused by repressed anger, stress, anxiety and sexual abuse.

Future historians of biology will be puzzled when they study the subject of obesity. They will scratch their heads looking for clues to why we chose to indulge in irrelevant discourses about the "psychological causes" of obesity when the simple facts of biology stared at us. They will not wonder about the causes of obesity and sluggishness of our tissues. They will wonder about the obesity and sluggishness of our intellects.

ON CRAVING ANGER

For optimal health, we need to clear the cortical clutter. We need to seek limbic openness. No one really knows enough to be a pessimist, so wrote Norman Cousins. To this I must add that *there is an absolute limit to how much a person can suffer.* In *The Cortical Monkey and Healing,* I wrote that there are three shapes of suffering: the suffering of the moment, the remembered suffering of the past, and the feared future suffering. Clearing the cortical clutter helps enormously in coping with the last two types of suffering.

The cortical monkey is a tenacious creature. It loves to argue. It calculates, competes, cautions and creates images of pain and anguish. It also sets us up for reverberating cycles of past hurts and feared future hurts. It has a voracious appetite for imagined suffering.

THE CORTICAL MONKEY LOVES TO RECYCLE MISERY

The cortical monkey loves to sit in judgment. It loves to censor. It thrives on criticism. When no one else is around, it thrives on self-criticism. It has an insatiable hunger for punishing thoughts. So we must recognize and reject its unending demands. We must approve of ourselves every morning and every hour of the day. And then every living moment, every breath.

It is a common clinical observation among clinical ecologists and physician-nutritionists that craving for a particular food, and allergy and reactivity to that food are flip sides of the same coin. In other words, we crave a food to seek relief from symptoms caused by its absence (withdrawal), just as a heroin addict craves for heroin to obtain relief from heroin withdrawal symptoms. We know that for both the food-reactive person and the heroin addict, such relief is temporary and perpetuates the addiction. I frequently observe this phenomenon among my patients with anger and hostility. They crave for anger and hostility. These "dys-emotions" bring temporary relief and are followed by a recurrence of the anger and hostility craving.

These cycles go on and on. Each passing thought fuels this cycle until the craving for anger and hostility paralyzes the individual.

BEYOND POSITIVE THINKING

We Americans seem to believe that we can clever-think our way out of all our problems. This is a simplistic notion when it comes to problems of anger, hostility and hate. Extensive clinical work has convinced me of the futility of this approach.

The true long-term answer to the problem of anger craving is to dissolve it with self-regulation and the language of silence. Clever thinking is not the true answer to the these problem; the language of silence and the state of "no-thinking" are. The best clinical results in my experience are obtained with methods of self-regulation which bring forth limbic openness through inner visceral energy changes.

What is the only part of the human condition which lies to us? Our thinking brain. Have I ever seen a heart or a muscle or a lung which lies? No. Indeed our body viscera never learned how to lie. Lying is the exclusive domain of our intellects. So why listen at all times to the only part of our human condition which lies? I would rather listen to all the other parts of my body which I know never lie to me. The body tissues can be only listened to with the "language of silence."

Limbic openness is a state beyond positive thinking, and the way to reach limbic openness is through the language of silence. However, there is often a real problem here. As one of my patients told me, autoregulation is like bank credit: The banks will not give us credit when we need it most. They will often throw their money at us when we do not need it. Progress in dissolving anger, hostility and hate is often painfully slow for those who need it most. Not everyone can move directly from anger craving to limbic openness. This is where meditation, affirmations and prayers are most valuable.

ON LEARNING TO BE HAPPY FOR OTHERS

Being happy for others is a powerful strategy for dissolving anger and hate. Initially it requires deliberate efforts. With time, it becomes a way of life. Anger is destructive. We all know this. Being happy for others is emancipating. We often do not recognize this. Being happy for others at one time may mean we feel good about what they may wear or own. But at another level, it is a spiritual dimension.

Angry people are generous in mind. They share their anger freely. They do it with those who they think need it as well as with those who may not. Anger, I wrote in *The Cortical Monkey and Healing*, is a molecular event. It lights up a thousand other anger molecules. Happiness is also a molecular event. It also lights up a thousand happiness molecules. This is not difficult to see or document today with suitable electrophysiological equipment.

What is the secret of success for organizations such as Alcoholics Anonymous and Recovery? People in these programs learn to be happy for each other. Each individual in turn "shares" his misery and anguish with the group. People in the group see how this "sharing of anguish" is liberating for that person. They are *happy* for him, and so the program moves on, from one person to the other. Each person learns to be happy for the others in the group. How often do they realize that it is through their *being* happy for others that their own spirits are lifted? I do not know. People become happy through the happiness of others.

I came here to see if someone here will kill my husband for me.

Sometime ago I was looking for a conference room in a hospital in New York City. I made a wrong turn, entered in a different conference room, and took a seat in the back. It was a meeting of Alcoholics Anonymous. It was my first contact with a group like that. People shared their hurts and anger. I was deeply moved by their courage, their strength in adversity, and ultimately their victory. People spoke when they wanted to. A woman next to me raised her arm. The discussion leader acknowledged her. She spoke, half in laughter, half in agony, "I am Shirley. I came here to see if someone will kill my husband for me. But I suppose no one here will do that for me."

The Shirleys of this world need the language of silence more than anything else. They need limbic openness more than anyone else. But anger and limbic openness are mutually exclusive. Limbic openness is not something people can order when they are hurt as badly as Shirley is. Shirley has to prepare herself for limbic openness, with patience, reflection, meditation, prayer, happiness for others and the language of silence.

I often hear that probing the wounds of the psyche is akin to a surgeon lancing an abscess. This seemed very cogent to me during my early years in surgery. I lanced an awful lot of abscesses in those years. After an abscess is opened and the pus let out, the wounds heals from below. I witnessed that on many an occasion. Does this hold for anger and hate? Is anger an abscess, waiting to be lanced by clever words of someone skillful in using words as lances? Is hatred a pool of putrid material, ripe for plucking out by someone with some great healing power implicit in his high credentials? As a surgeon and a pathologist, I never faced such questions about these popular notions of health and disease. My patients have forced me to think differently. *The cortical monkey loves to recycle misery. The language of silence heals.* That is what my angry patients with deep reservoirs of hate have taught me.

Several thoughts crossed my mind in the AA meeting. It occurred to me that we physicians could learn many things from that group. In an AA meeting, the essence of the meeting is *listening.* Our medical meetings are different. We physicians love verbal war games. One physician proudly declares that drug ABC is the *treatment of choice* for XYZ disease while he is shouted down by another who pronounces, with overriding authority, that the real treatment of choice for this disease is the surgical procedure his mentor developed at the university hospital where he trained. How often do I sit in these meetings wondering why the treatment of choice for every suffering has to be a drug or a surgical procedure? I wonder why no one thinks the treatment of choice for any patient can be listening, learning, understanding and *knowing* the cause of his affliction.

Returning to the subject of the role of anger and hostility in the cause of obesity and ill-health, my thoughts turn to human need for kindness and love. Anger and hate, it seems to me, are the flip sides of the coins of kindness and love. At present, love is a taboo subject in medicine. In the words of my friend, Choua, kindness as a healing tool in medicine is equally irrelevant to practitioners of N^2D^2 medicine as they fight with diseases and among themselves for patients who suffer from diseases.

Hate, as a relation to objects is older than love. It derives from the narcissistic ego's primordial repudiation of the external world with its outpouring of stimuli."

Sigmund Freud
in *Instincts and their vicissitudes* S.E., vol 14

Freud was an astute observer of human nature. I do not fully know the circumstances and evidence which led Freud to make the preceding statement. My own clinical experience has been different, and so is my perception of the twin problems of hate and anger. That hate and anger create a state of *dis-ease* and lead to disease, I have no doubt. That hate as a relation to objects is older than love, that does not seem true to me.

I close this chapter with the words with which I ended *The Cortical Monkey and Healing.*

It seems improbable that man will ever fully understand the healing energy of love, or to be more precise, the healing energy of God. Medical technology, itself an expression of God's energy, is beginning to allow us to measure some things about love, and then reproduce them. Measurements and reproducibility make up the language of science. One day, it seems to me, the men of medicine and men of spirits will meet at some summit of union. The energy of love will have brought them together.

A Gift For Every Moment

There is a sculptor in the sky with a gift for every moment. Look up with the language of silence, receive the gift and treasure it.

From *The Limbic Dog and Directed Pulses*

Chapter 6

Why Dieting Does Not Work

Dieting Does Not Work

People do lose weight with dieting programs, at least on a short-term basis. This happens largely because of the loss of water and muscle, conditions which threaten our long-term health. People who do lose weight with dieting gain it back, in most cases even when they continue to diet.

Dieting does not work. We know this by common experience. We also know this from the study of molecular dynamics in human biology. Dieting is not the answer if our goals are good health with a lean, energetic body. We know this by sheer intuition. Notwithstanding the enormous advertising pressure on us Americans to the contrary, it is a hard scientific fact that dieting is not good for one's health from a life span perspective.

The dieting industry spends enormous sums of money in commercials trying to convince people that their dieting products work. They often show men and women with lithesome bodies giving dazzling testimonials to the value of their "balanced" diets, their frozen foods, their liquid diets, and their behavior modification techniques based on their favorite concepts of neurophysiology, neuropsychology, and neurobiology. The results of meticulous studies performed with sound methods of research tell a different story altogether.

There are over one hundred young men and women who work in our hospital laboratory and several hundred more who work in other departments of the hospital. Over the years I have watched many of them go through cycles of losing weight with diets and then gaining it back, usually ending up with more pounds than when they started.

There have been some exceptions. Some people read a lot about nutrition, learn to select their foods carefully, change their eating habits, put themselves on regular exercise, lose weight and keep themselves slim and vigorous. The term catabolic principle will be foreign to them, the concept of the catabolic maladaptation unknown. The elements of mitochondrial health, enzymatic efficiency, aging-oxidant and life span foods, cortical sugar-burning and limbic fat-burning exercises would be unfamiliar to them. They probably would not even know the basic aspects of the structure and function of the myocyte (muscle cell) and the adipocyte (fat cell). Yet these people were unwittingly (and successfully) applying the principles of the catabolic principle.

What does the scientific literature say about experience with the weight loss programs? It almost uniformly gives us a dismal picture.

... the results of this study, the first controlled trial of very low calorie diets confirm the widespread belief that rapid weight loss is followed by almost equally rapid regain.

J Consult Clin Psychology 54:482; 1986.

The literature has not shown the combination of drugs and behavior therapy to be very promising.

Obesity:Basic Aspects and Clinical Application. Med Clin N America Jan 89 pg 17

The issue is not whether or not people lose weight with dieting. Ask veteran dieters. They have lost and gained weight dozens of times. They will read this and readily see the plight of the butterfly. With dieting, people lose weight by losing water, muscle, some fats (as well as energy and vigor). This is entirely predictable. Dieting starves tissues and their cells. Dieting dehydrates. Dieting tires. Research in the pathophysiology of dieting has clearly shown the many health hazards of dieting.

With dieting, we lose muscle. The dieters must remember that the heart is a muscle organ. Rapid loss of heart muscle, as a part of rapid initial weight loss obtained with the dieting programs, can be dangerous for the heart. Indeed, death in several young dieters has been attributed to the effects of dieting on the heart in many carefully studied cases. The mercenaries of dieting will not teach us about these dangers of dieting.

Demonstration that VLCDs (very low calorie diets) containing predominantly protein diminished the negative nitrogen balance associated with starvation rapidly led to popularity of these diets. ...... The attendant publicity encouraged thousands of Americans to go on this diet, many using the regimen as a sole source of nutrition.

Deaths in people on this diet began to be reported to the FDA and the collagen preparations were restricted by the FDA. Sours and Isner and their coworkers published a survey of 58 deaths, 17 of whom had no apparent complicating features other than adherence to the diet."

Med Clin N America Jan 1989 pg 209

Overweight and obese people know their suffering. They feel tired. They often resent the way they look. They want help and are willing to pay for it. Merchants of the dieting industry know there is a lot of money to be made with the promises of slimness. They do not see the anguish of dieting and hurt of regaining the lost weight along with some dividend pounds. The only thing important to them is that their packaged foods and lies bring them riches.

Soon thereafter, the Cambridge Diet was introduced into this country and, at its peak, generated revenues at a rate of $500 million per year. A report to the FDA noted that approximately 5 million people used the Cambridge Diet. The lack of health professional supervision and several highly publicized deaths led to condemnation of the Cambridge Diet and VLCDs in general.

Med Clin N America Jan 1989 pg 210

So some people gained riches. Some others lost their lives.

How does dieting adversely affect the structure and function of the heart? I indicated earlier that dieters lose water and muscle before they lose fat. The heart is a muscular organ and suffers from this loss. The more rapid the weight loss, the higher the risk of heart complications from muscle loss. The stress of dieting predictably increases oxidant damage to the heart muscle. Packed dieting formulas generally are rich in oxidized foods and further increase oxidant injury. The heart comes under a double jeopardy: oxidant load on it increases substantially, and its capacity to sustain the oxidant injury decreases significantly. How does an injured heart express its hurt? By palpitating and beating with irregular rhythm. I cite below one such study.

... found cardiac arrhythmias on Holter monitoring in subjects on VLCD (very low calorie diet) with hydrolyzed collagen, but no arrhythmias when the protein source was of high quality.

Med Clin N America, Jan. 1989 pg 211

What is not readily apparent from such reports is the enormous health damage caused by diets. Dieting, as I discussed in the section *On the Nature of Obesity,* leads to emaciation of muscle cells, bloating of fat cells, accumulation of toxic fats in tissues, sluggishness of enzymes, and fatigue. Beyond this is the untold misery caused by dieting. Hopes of obese people are raised and dashed. They lose weight and regain it, usually ending up somewhat heavier than they were before they started their diet.

Few professionals in health care have benefitted so much from their own ignorance and incompetence than those in the business of dieting. Few professionals have hurt those who trust them with their health more than those employed by the dieting industry.

Dieting does not work for several reasons.

Dieting Is Illogical From A Metabolic Standpoint

Obesity is a catabolic maladaptation. The essential defect

in this maladaptation is that fat-burning enzymes in the muscle mitochondria are sluggish and fat cells are bloated with fats, often of a toxic nature.

In the body, sugars and amino acids are converted into fats for storage. But this conversion occurs in only one direction. Fats cannot be converted back into sugars or proteins. There is only one way bloated fat cells can rid themselves of fats: by using ("burning") the fat for energy generation in muscles. It follows that the only way for obese people to lose fat is by increasing their muscle mass, sharpening their lipolytic (fat-burning) enzymes, and increasing the rate of burning fat. This cannot be done by starving the muscles and their enzymes. Dieting is exactly the wrong thing to do.

Dieting Is Inappropriate
From the Food Allergy Standpoint

Food incompatibility, in my experience, is the single most common cause of undue fatigue. Mold allergy is next in order of importance. Both food and mold allergies can contribute to the problem of obesity, directly by inducing allergic reactions that cause fatigue and indirectly by facilitating the destructive capacity of aging-oxidant molecules.

Food allergy is of two types: Fixed food allergy and cyclic food allergy. Fixed food allergy causes a reaction each time the specific allergic food is eaten. For example, a person with shrimp allergy develops hives after eating shrimp every time. Similarly, a patient with milk asthma develops a wheezing attack each time he drinks milk or has some dairy products. Cyclic food allergy does not always cause demonstrable reactions after each food exposure. Further reactions may be immediate or be delayed for several hours. One of my associates can eat chicken twice a week without symptoms. She develops symptoms if she eats chicken three or more times a week.

Food allergy requires suitable tests for diagnosis. The popular dieting programs almost always ignore this important aspect. I discuss the subject of food allergy tests in the chapter *On Limbic Eating.*

Dieting Is Ill-Advised From the Standpoint of Chronic Illness

Obese people often suffer from several types of bowel ailments. Many of these ailments are related to problems of altered bowel transit time (constipation with episodes of diarrhea), increased bowel permeability (the so-called Leaky Gut Syndrome), digestive diseases and absorptive dysfunctions, altered bowel flora and yeast overgrowth, and parasitic infestations. I discuss these critically important issues at length in my monograph *The Altered Bowel Ecology States and Health Preservation.*

Many overweight and obese people suffer from chronic fatigue, headaches, sleep disorders, anxiety and stress, PMS, high blood pressure, heart disease, vascular insufficiency, muscle cramps due to mineral deficiencies, arthritis, joint and ligament disorders. Dieting frequently worsens these disorders. Most dieting programs completely ignore these co-existing problems, often to the detriment of the general health of the individual. Proper management of these disorders is essential for a successful program for weight loss and promotion of health for the life span of the individual.

Dieting Is Irrational From a Hunger and Satiety Standpoint

Hunger and satiety signals are important biological cues. They must be heeded if we hope to remain healthy and energetic for any period of time. The very foundation of the dieting programs is based on negation or denial of these essential biologic signals.

Why did nature create satiety signals? This question arose in my mind one day while I was reading one weight expert's ideas of a very low fat diet? It is common observation that a meal of vegetables and fruits leaves us hungry within an hour or less. Meals with some substance to them require some fats. If fats were really as bad as the high priests of drug medicine tell us they are, why would nature assign them such a central role in hunger signals? Why hunger for something that is not necessary? I found the answer some days later during my limbic run. The need for fats for satiety must be linked to the health of plasma membranes. The plasma membranes (membranes covering the cells and their organelles) are essentially made up of fats. These membranes, I wrote in the chapter On the Nature of Obesity, separate an inner order within the cell from an external disorder. They are the gatekeepers. They are also the first targets of oxidant molecules. Nature built them of fats, and made fats essential for satiety to assure a continued supply of raw material for their maintenance and repair work. Do the experts of very-low-fat diets ever reflect on the inner workings of cells? Do they ever ponder over such marvels of biology?

Fats are essential for cellular health. Fats are essential for a healthy life span. *What we do not need is oxidized fats. I discuss this subject at some length in my monograph Choua, Cholesterol Cats and Chelation.*

Dieting Is Ill-advised From the Standpoint of Injured and Oxidized Foods

From a life span perspective, I wrote earlier, I divide foods into two basic groups of life span foods and aging-oxidant foods. Life span foods support and sustain life span molecules. Injured and oxidized foods favor aging-oxidant molecules. Obesity, premature aging, degenerative diseases are, in a large measure, the consequences of aging-oxidant foods. I discuss this subject at length in the chapter *Life Span Food Choices.*

Dieting Is Ill-conceived From a Life Span Standpoint

Dieting is a quick-fix approach which almost always fails and frequently causes severe metabolic disorders including muscle disorders, liver injury, gall bladder disorders, and even death. In my clinical work, I have always had a strong commitment to the issue of the life span. I strongly resist all those "strategies" which can give me good initial results and poor long-term results. Dieting focuses on weight loss. The Catabolic Principle focuses on optimal health and a lean, energetic body for the length of the expected life span.

What are the stories of the veteran dieters? These are stories of dieting and deprivation, of dashed hopes and disillusionment, of distrust and disbelief. Ask them. These are accounts of tired bodies and bruised spirits. The annals of dieting programs are replete with stories of people with serious weight problems who eat little but do not lose weight. There are people who will lose some weight initially on a limited caloric intake and then gain back their lost weight even when they stay on the starvation levels of restricted diets. I discuss this subject in the chapter *The Catabolic Principle.*

HUNGER SIGNALS AND DIETING

It is a widely held, and in my judgement, mistaken belief that hunger is a signal from a collection of nerve cell in a part of the brain called the hypothalamus. This belief is based upon some rat experiments that showed that the destruction of some neurones (nerve cells in the ventromedial portion of the hypothalamus in the brain) causes the rat to overeat and become obese. Evidence from subsequent experiments strongly opposed such simplistic notions. Specifically, after some initial weight gain, the rats do not overeat even when encouraged to do so, and do not gain additional weight (see the section *On the Nature of Obesity*).

It seems to me that the physiology of hunger can be understood only through molecular thinking about events which occur *at the level of fat and muscle cells* and not in the brain. How do cells *at the site of action* talk to each other? How do enzymes sense the availability of food and respond to them? How do arteries in different parts of the body open up with self-regulatory methods such as directed pulses? I describe this method in detail in my booklet *Directed Pulses*. How does a patient in the throes of an asthma attack allow his bronchial tubes to open up without drugs so he can breathe? How does an overactive thyroid gland return back to health without drugs? How do abnormal thyroid chemistry tests become normal in such a person? I have observed too many molecular and cellular events like this to enumerate here. The essential point here is that the tissues *know* what is the right thing to do only if we let them.

My personal clinical observations are consistent with the concepts of the emerging field of auto-organization in biology that I alluded to in the chapter On the Nature of Obesity. Auto-organization, in essence, is the phenomenon in which electrons and molecules demonstrate an innate ability to organize themselves in form and function which is necessary for the structural and functional integrity and the total health of the whole organism. Evolution in biology is then seen as a natural order of things in which natural selection occurs in living organisms during an unending process of electron, molecular and cellular auto-organization.

I include this passing reference to auto-organization in biology to provide scientific support for my viewpoint that the phenomenon of hunger has much more to do with the function of the myocyte, the adipocyte, the liver cell, and the cells of other body organs rather than the simplistic belief that it is an exclusive domain of the hypothalamus. There are simply too many holes in this hypothalamus story. For example, why do the cells of the pancreas put out more insulin when the fat cells begin to accumulate extra fat? Why do the bloated fat cells fight so hard to maintain status quo, even when the obese person puts himself on a near starvation diet? Why do muscle cells offer themselves as sacrificial lambs when a person begins to diet? Why do fat cells of the rat collect excessive fat when the rat's hypothalamus is cooked with electrodes? And why do the fat cells of the rat refuse to continue to accumulate more fat after the initial fat gain in the hypothalamus cooking experiments?

Where do the hunger signals of children raised on a diet of greasy cheese burgers, french fries, milk shakes and cookies fit in the natural order of things? The answer: nowhere. These unfortunate children are victims of marketing moguls of our fast food industry. Their parents are often innocent parents, their physicians generally ignorant about all essential issues in human nutrition. Few things are as saddening as listening to pediatricians who trivialize the health hazards of toxic foods. Little do they realize they are accomplices in food crimes against our children, by default if not by design.

Dollar an Hour to Keep the Kid Away.

Sometimes ago I had lunch in the hospital cafeteria with some colleagues. A pediatrician was talking about his day at the pool with his children. He described how frustrated he became with his children until he thought of an ingenious plan to bring peace to his family. He gave them each a dollar for ice cream every hour they were at the pool. A small price to pay for peace! he exclaimed.

At another occasion, one of the internists on our staff talked about taking his children to a hamburger outlet for a quick dinner. I don't know what these nutritionists are fussing about, he said. It all ends up in the stomach anyway. On days like these I simply eat my lunch and return to the laboratory. I suppose drugs and nutrition do not mix well.

LIPASES, THE GATEKEEPER ENZYMES

How long have the dieting experts been around? How long have lipases been around?

These questions may seem frivolous. For serious students of biology and people interested in optimal health, however, these are essential questions. A search for answers to questions like these leads us to enduring truths in biology.

Lipases are gatekeeper enzymes for the adipocytes and

they represent molecules that regulate how much fat enters fat cells and how much leaves them. Nature has given them some important assignments. The primary duties of these enzymes are to prevent cell death by starvation.

These enzymes have been around for millions of years. They were given the responsibility for saving living things from starvation long before America became the breadbasket for the whole world (and poisoned its soil with synthetic chemicals in pursuit of greater profits). Man had not thought of storing grains in silos yet. Refrigerators had not been invented yet. It is important to recognize that the lipases still do not know about these changes. Lipases still do not know when and from where the next meal will come. How will they receive their next shipment of nourishment. Our enzymes have not learned yet that there are such things as food stamps. During the hunting-gathering epoch, long before man learned to farm and store food, lipase enzymes *knew* that they could not *plan* their activities. Between the feasts there would be famine; lipases *knew* that. They had to be ever prepared for conservation. That is what the lipases do. When the food is available in abundance, lipases hoard food, and store it as fat in the fat cells. When the food is not available during dieting, the lipases *sense* an impending famine. They respond quickly. They hoard yet more food as fat. The dieters get hurt both ways, when he eats and when he does not eat.

Go Ahead! Starve Us,
Lipases Taunt the Dieting Experts

Lipases do not have much respect for our dieting experts

and their silly notions of metabolism and health. When they are threatened with starvation (that is how these enzymes perceive dieting), they go in high gear. They tenaciously latch on to fat. You want to starve us? Lipases mock the dieting experts. Go ahead, try something else, they dare the dieting experts. You want to lose weight by starving us? Tough! You want to crumble our homes (the fat cells are homes to lipases), we will crumble you. You want to lose pounds? Silly! go lose them in muscles.

Hunger to me is an essential signal from myocytes, adipocytes, liver cells and the cells of other body organs. Hunger is essential for cellular health. Denying hunger is being deaf to the needs of billions of individual cells. How long can a person do that without putting in jeopardy the health of the whole organism? I might ask another question here. How does a person become obese in the first place? By playing deaf to energy, molecular and cellular signals. How can we hope to reverse a problem caused by ignoring one set of signals by a deliberate plan to ignore another set of signals? When the dieter starves, he receives many cellular catabolic signals. When he gorges, he receives other signals from a stomach and a bowel in distress. There are yet other signals from the heart and other body organs which the dieter is too exhausted to perceive. Recent research has shown that cyclical weight losses and weight gains have clear detrimental effects on the heart.

Eating, Insulin and Lipases

It is a common error among people (and many professionals) to associate blood and tissue fats with fat in foods, and to link sugars in the food with blood and tissue levels of insulin. Such "compartmentalized" thinking is used to promote whatever suite the whims of dieting experts. This would appear to be a simplistic notion even from a basic standpoint of the *holistic relatedness in human biology*. Indeed, there is a large body of clinical and experimental data which refute such simplistic notions.

Lipases clear plasma of triglyceride-rich lipoproteins. These enzymes also generate free fatty acids from these blood lipids and store them in fat cells. Post-prandial states (the states of metabolism after eating) are associated with higher levels of insulin. Insulin enhances the activity, speeds up the rate of synthesis of lipases, and increases *m*RNA, the messenger molecules which promote the production of these enzymes in the tissue. (*J Bio Chem 264:3177, 1989)*

There are other costs of ignored catabolic signals. There are molecular events which cause anger and hostility. There are raised hopes and dashed hopes. There is the guilt of bingeing, and the hurt of failure. There is anxiety and depression. Dieting does not trigger panic attacks, but it often compounds the problem. Indeed, my nutritional approach to the prevention of panic attacks is directed at regulating the molecular energy pathways and preventing molecular roller coasters.

WHY DO WE EAT?

To sublimate hostility? To dissipate suppressed anger?

To cope with the consequences of childhood abuse? To defy a boss? To resolve co-dependency? To cope with abandonment? To repair a disintegrated personality? To express subliminal anxiety? Next time you see a thin person eat a large meal, ask him which one of the above applies to him.

Why does a thin person overeat? Why does an obese person overeat? Both eat because they are hungry. An obese person carries some additional burdens. He suffers from catabolic maladaptation. At each meal he encounters a maladaptive metabolism, some enzymes sluggish from disuse, some injured by oxidized foods and some poisoned by designer killer molecules of antibiotics, pesticides and fungicides. When an obese person eats, he is also responding to a "catabolic call." Could it be something simple like that? Could it be a simple signal of hunger distorted by a catabolic maladaptation? An abnormal hunger signal, but a hunger signal nonetheless? Of course stress, anxiety, panic and depression increase the burdens on an already burdened catabolic status. But these factors do not cause obesity. Obesity is catabolic maladaptation.

We concoct ingenious theories to hide our ignorance of the simple facts of biology. Why does an overweight person overeat, we love to ask? It must be to cope with his anger, we hasten to enlighten him? Or to get even with someone, our imagination soars. Or because he is rebelling, we bring out our psychoanalytic tools. Or because it is a rainy day. Or because it is a clear balmy day. Or because it is vacation time.

When an obese person overeats, we are told, he is driven by anger or hostility or depression. But what drives the thin person when he overeats? Anger, anxiety, hostility or depression? How is it that anger and depression pump fat into fat cells of only obese people? Why don't they do the same to the fat cells of the thin person? The gurus of the dieting industry do not like to address these questions.

Hunger signals do not call for denial of dieting. These signals call for life-sustaining, lifespan foods. The essential issues here are unoxidized foods and up-regulation of fat-burning enzymes with slow and sustained exercises.

EAT-LITTLE AND EAT-VERY-LITTLE THEORIES OF DIETING

Many diets have been proposed as solutions to the problem of obesity. Indeed, the number of such diets is a tribute to the ingenuity of people who sell diets and diet products. In general, the less rational the diets, the more flashy their names. For many people, dieting is a bad word. It brings back to them bad memories of false promises, disappointments, and yes, sometimes outright deception.

Following, I give a brief summary of some of the popular diets and their disadvantages. I include a description of many of the serious health hazards of these diets at the end of this section.

Dieting by common use means eating less. Implicit in this statement is the theory that if only we could eat less, we will become thin and healthy. There are two broad theories which the merchants of dieting promote: 1) eat less; and 2) eat very little, if at all.

Diets based on both the eat less and the eat-little, if-at-all theories can be further subdivided into two categories: 1) eat less of balanced foods category; and 2) eat less by eating only one type of food category.

BALANCED REDUCING DIETS

The proponents of this diet advise us to eat small portions of everything.

These experts, professionals or otherwise, generally understand neither the true nature of obesity nor the toxic or allergic potential of any of the common foods. They are unburdened by any knowledge of nutrition, metabolism, exercise physiology, human ecology, or catabolic maladaptation.

Sometimes they advise us to eat slowly (good advice for improving digestion, but surely an overweight person can eat an awful lot of food slowly). At other times they advise us to leave some food on the plate (overweight people find this advice quite acceptable. They simply load the plate more heavily). Other advice includes "putting the fork down between morsels", "imaging themselves in bikinis when eating", and "directing imagery at their hypothalamic set point."

Eating less seems to be the simple answer to the complex problem of obesity for promoters of such diets.

MONO-FOOD DIETS

Merchants of the mono-food diets have even a more fascinating theory to support their diets. The theory behind the so-called one-food diets is that the person will soon get bored with the monotony of a diet composed of a single food. Some such diets do allow occasional use of other foods but not enough to prevent sheer boredom. Boredom, after all is the primary strategy behind such diets. Regardless how good the food, eating a single food eventually means less eating. It amazes me that some professionals could seriously impose such an absurdity upon anyone. It is equally amazing that some people would accept such advice.

Perhaps the most amusing of mono-food diets is the ice cream diet. It must have been conceived by someone who both loved and hated ice cream.

The rice diet was originally proposed in 1949 by Kempner for the treatment of heart and kidney diseases (Ann Int Med 31:821; 1949). It soon became a popular weight loss diet. The practitioners of this diet try to subsist on white rice. A rice diet is an excellent way to experimentally produce a vitamin and mineral deficiency syndrome, as are all other single-food diets.

PROTEIN DIETS

There is a plethora of such diets. Most of these diets are liquid formulas composed of proteins, carbohydrates, vitamins and minerals. These diets are attractive because they save us from the labor of deciding what to eat and, of course, they save time. I wonder what it is that we do with the time so saved.

As a part of a complete program that addresses all the causes that lead to catabolic maladaptation as described in this book, formulas composed of amino acids, peptides (short chains of amino acids) and proteins are indeed of considerable help. But this is rarely done. The common practice is to look at protein drinks as the real solution to the problem of obesity.

KETOGENIC DIETS

Ketone bodies are actually three chemicals which are formed when fat is incompletely catabolized in the body. The three chemicals are ketone, acetoacetic acid, and hydroxybutyric acid. Of these ketone cannot be further broken down in the body.

Ketogenic diets permit liberal amounts of commonly used fats and proteins. The carbohydrates are either severely limited or eliminated altogether. Such diets are expected to lead to ketonuria. Some such diets actually encourage the practitioner to test the urine and make certain that ketosis does exist.

The term ketosis refers to the abnormal collection of ketone bodies in the tissues and blood. Ketone bodies are formed when fat is incompletely catabolized. Ketone bodies are often seen in the urine (ketonuria) of infants and children in toxic states accompanied by vomiting and diarrhea. The dangers of accumulation of excess ketone bodies are well described in medical texts.

Diabetic Ketonuria. The presence of ketonuria indicates the presence of ketoacidosis (ketosis) and may provide a warning of impending coma.

Clinical Diagnosis and Management by Laboratory Methods W.B. Saunders Company Philadelphia 1984, Page 413

It is well established that ketogenic diets can lead to weight loss. Most individuals rapidly regain all lost weight as soon as they return to normal eating.

From a life span perspective, ketosis (and excess of acidity in the body which it inevitably causes), is not a sound strategy.

EAT-LITTLE-IF-ANY DIETS

These are truly dangerous diets. The more obese the person, the more damaging the diet.

Self-imposed starvation has been tried by many dieters. The results are uniformly dismal. The dieter-starver loses weight rapidly during the initial phases. These false hopes are dashed within weeks as continued starvation causes progressive irritability and lack of energy but no additional weight loss.

We conclude that weight loss in very obese subjects leads to increased activity and expression of lipoprotein lipase, thereby potentially enhancing lipid storage and making further weight loss more difficult.

N Eng J Med 322:1053; 1990

Starvation causes problems of mood, memory and mentation. Fat cells are quite resistant to starvation. They hold onto their fat well as muscle tissue is broken down for the essential energy requirements of life. Next follow bad breath, headaches, muscle cramps, constipation (and diarrhea for some), hair loss, dry skin, menstrual irregularities, lost interest in sex, heart palpitations and nervous tremors. During starvation, the classical teaching in physiology holds, the energy requirements initially call up glycogen reserves in the liver. Glycogen is converted into glucose for utilization by brain, heart and other body organs. When glycogen reserves are depleted, the energy enzymes next call on protein reserves in muscle, heart, kidney and other body organs. If the starving person still ignores the visceral (limbic) messages from his tissues, the next change is ketosis. The accumulation of ketone bodies (small fragments of incompletely broken down fats) increases acidotic and oxidant stress on plasma membranes. All these changes cause ill health. None of these changes can reverse the catabolic maladaptation that is the root cause of obesity.

Recent studies have challenged some old "established" knowledge of the physiology of starvation. Specifically, there is a widespread belief that proteins in muscle and other tissues are initially spared during starvation while glycogen in the liver is converted to glucose to meet the energy requirements. This viewpoint has been proven to be inaccurate by recent studies performed with magnetic resonance spectroscopy. It is clear now that muscle tissue begins to be cannibalized as soon as starvation begins.

The surprising observation in this study was the calculated net rate of hepatic glycogenolysis for the first 22 h of fasting, which accounted for only 36% of total glucose production (range 19-54%), while gluconeogenesis accounted for 64%.

Lancet 339:152; 1992.

How is this bit of medical jargon translated in common language? Tissue breakdown for energy release begins as soon as starvation begins and occurs at a much higher rate than was previously believed. The lesson for the dieter is abundantly clear: Prepare to lose muscle and vitality as soon as you begin dieting .

ADVERSE EFFECTS OF DIETING

There is a long list of medical reports of serious adverse effects of dieting. The health hazards of dieting affect all body organs. Before I discuss many of the well known ill-effects of dieting, I want to comment on the one which is closest to my heart.

Dieting causes anger. Anger produces potent oxidizing molecules. Oxidizing molecules injure fat-burning enzymes. Injured fat-burning enzymes lead to yet more fat accumulation. The vicious cycle goes on.

Following is a listing of well documented adverse effects of dieting.

General: Dehydration, lethargy, undue tiredness, persistent fatigue, excessive sensitivity to cold, decreased physical stamina, excessive hair loss, dry skin, halitosis, and electrolyte imbalance. **Nervous System:** Weakness, mood and memory difficulties, irritability, headache, light-headedness, and inability to concentrate. **Gastrointestinal:** Abdominal discomfort and bloating, nausea, vomiting, constipation, episodes of diarrhea, fatty change of the liver, and exacerbations of gall bladder disease. **Genitourinary:** Menstrual irregularities (abnormal cycles, heavy, prolonged bleeding as well as minimal bleeding), loss of libido, and increased tendency of kidney stones. **Cardiovascular:** Irregular heart beats(arrhythmias), palpitation, postural hypotension (low blood pressure on stooping down), and myocardial atrophy (loss of heart muscle). There are other serious long-term adverse effects of dieting and cyclical fluctuations in weight. In one study, the 25-year crude risk of coronary death was 26% in a group of people who went through cycles of weight loss and weight gain, 15% in a group of people who gained weight but did not lose it with dieting and 14% in the "no change in weight group."

Sudden Death

The risk of sudden cardiac death from causes related to dieting is not mere rhetoric. I referred earlier in the chapter to a survey of 58 deaths, 17 of whom had no apparent complicating features other than adherence to the diet. These young people were dieting and died suddenly. No specific cause of death was found at autopsy. The pathologists performing the autopsy and clinicians who attended upon these inand chemical ividuals before death concluded that the likely ause of death was electrophysiologic and chemical changes associated with dieting.

The skylight stays; the butterfly dies.

Chapter 7

The
Catabolic Principle

For good health for the full human life span, we need to eat sparingly. The ancients knew this empirically; we are learning it from our animal experiments.

In catabolic maladaptation, however, the simple strategy of eating less — reduced caloric intake with dieting — almost never works. The basic problem in catabolic maladaptation, I wrote earlier, is down-regulation of fat-burning enzymes caused by oxidized, denatured foods and environmental pollutants, and down-regulation of muscle enzymes caused by inactivity. For weight loss with reversal of catabolic maladaptation, both issues must be addressed, concurrently and with equal emphasis. Energy enzymes cannot be up-regulated without more food. The idea of eating more food to lose weight creates a paradox, a skylight of illusion, for those who have not studied human energy dynamics and metabolism.

The catabolic principle is the principle of eating *more* food and doing *more* excise to *lose* body fat by increasing the efficiency of fat-burning enzymes. The clinical application of this principal must be closely supervised by a knowledgeable and experienced professional.

I briefly wrote in the preface of this book about the intuitive insights of the ancients into matters of human metabolism and health. They recognized that the metabolism can be slowed down with fasting. They advised fasting for periods of silence, meditation and prayer. They also knew metabolism can be speeded up with eating and physical activity. The concept of the catabolic principal evolved in my mind as I observed some people gain weight as they ate less with dieting. In many cases, my patients lost some weight initially as they reduced their caloric intake and then gained the lost pounds, usually with some additional pounds, *even though they continued to eat at the reduced rate.* Next, they further reduced their food intake. Again they lost some weight initially only to regain it back while they maintained their reduced caloric intake. After each initiative, they ended up with less food and more body fat. This apparent paradox puzzled me initially. On deeper reflection I recognized how fully consistent my clinical observations were with the intuitive wisdom of the ancients.

OBESITY IS FATTENING
CAN SLIMNESS BE SLIMMING?

Some recent studies conclusively prove that fat-burning enzymes in fat cells decrease in quantity and become less efficient as excess fat accumulates in the cells. In other words, *obesity in and of itself is fattening.* If obesity is fattening, could slimness be slimming? This seemed logical to me. But was it true? I wondered. Doing fat biopsies just to prove this point seemed grossly unfair to those whose flesh would have to be cut into just to satisfy my scientific curiosity. In all my previous research, I had had the good fortune not to inflict injury upon anyone merely to satisfy my intellectual interests. I realized, of course, this was not a difficult goal in research for a pathologist. Others may not be able to hold themselves to this ideal. As for me, I felt a strong visceral resistance to research in preventive medicine with invasive, tissue-cutting procedures. How else could I attack this problem? I wondered.

A simple solution arose in my mind. Why not experiment with my own body weight? During my early years in clinical medicine, my weight used to fluctuate between 142 and 146 pounds. Before I got interested in preventive medicine, I was, like most of my colleagues in medicine, interested only in diseases. Health was of no great interest to me. Fully immersed in my hospital laboratory work and in my research in immunology and pathology, I had allowed my weight to climb up all the way to 169 pounds. After I became interested in health rather than disease, and even before I finished *The cortical Monkey and Healing,* I had a blueprint of an exercise book in my mind. I had a vague notion that to write about exercise I needed to study the effects of different types of exercises upon myself. My ideas of the principles and practice of limbic exercise had not evolved in my mind yet. How to go about proving that slimness is indeed slimming was one of the many questions in my mind. I did have a sense that this question, like many others before it, would also resolve itself as I continued my work. So I began my experiments with exercise that I describe in *The Ghoraa and Limbic Exercise* and by eating different foods in varying amounts. I also experimented with both life span and aging-oxidant foods.

Some other observations in my clinical work with immune disorders also helped me think more clearly about the relationship between eating, slimming, dieting and gaining weight. I regularly test my patients with an electrodermal conductance technology for food incompatibilities. This technology offers a much broader perspective on the relationship of food to the human condition than the prevailing, and very narrow, views of food allergy. When I see them first, most of these patients eat the typical supermarket foods and are subject to frequent metabolic roller coasters. After doing food compatibility profiles, it usually takes them several weeks to move from the concept of dieting-food exclusion to a nutritional philosophy based on the inclusion of healthful foods at mealtime. It is at this stage that they begin to get a sense for *limbic listening* to their hunger signals as well as for the difference between life span foods and aging-oxidant foods and their effects on the detoxification enzymes. They begin to perform limbic exercise, and it is then that they begin to *know* the difference between up-regulated and down-regulated energy and detoxification enzymes.

Foods fuels the furnace of metabolism;
exercise stokes its fires.

In the clinical application of the catabolic principal, the element of eating more life span foods must be preceded by doing more fat-burning exercise. Furthermore, I stress that the beginner must follow the strategy of eating *more* to lose weight under close supervision of someone knowledgeable and experienced in matters of nutrition, metabolism and the difference between sugar-burning and fat-burning exercises. In the chapter Life Span Food Choices and in *The Ghoraa and Limbic Exercise*, I make specific recommendations for effective fat-burning exercise and sound nutritional philosophy. The general as well as professional readers should have no difficulty understanding the principles and practice of limbic exercise and limbic eating. In the appendix, I include addresses of the American Academy of Environmental Medicine and the American College for Advancement in Medicine. Physicians

who belong to these two organizations, in general, are
knowledgeable in these areas and are able to provide the
necessary professional guidance.

What is Catabolism?

Living organisms live by metabolism. The term
metabolism refers to all life processes that living organisms use
to turn chemical bond energy of foods into other forms of
energy—thermal energy for keeping the body warm,
electrochemical energy for building molecules, catabolic energy
for breaking molecules down and mechanical energy for
movements and work. The basic equation of metabolism has
two sides: 1) anabolism for building molecules, cells and tissues;
and 2) catabolism for breaking down molecules, cells and
tissues. The purpose of catabolism is to produce energy for
molecular repair and renewal. Health can be preserved, and life
span weight attained and maintained, only through balance and
harmony among molecules, cells and tissues. If the anabolic side
of this basic equation of life is put in jeopardy, human
development fails. If the catabolic side fails, our molecules
stagnate, our cells bloat, and our tissues decay. In essence, we
suffocate.

My working definition of the catabolic principle
emphasizes the following four elements:

First,

An overweight or obese person must *eat* more food, and

not less food as is   the conventional wisdom among the merchants of the dieting industry. He must do so under close professional supervision.

Overweight and obese people gain weight even when they cut down vigorously on their caloric intake. This occurs because catabolic efficiency falls when an overweight person diets and eats less. Initially, overweight people lose weight with diet programs that severely limit eating. As these people lose weight they also lose catabolic efficiency of enzymes in their fat cells. Within weeks their new weight is stabilized and further weight loss does not occur even if they cut down further on eating. Within weeks the person begins to gain weight *even as he keeps dieting.* Muscles can only be built with proteins consumed with food. More muscle can only be built by eating more and taking in more proteins. Muscles cannot be built from fats. The notion that an obese person can burn his fat and at the same time build his muscles from the energy released by burning fat is silly. Fat is regularly built from sugars and proteins. This is the way body stores extra calories for what it sees as possible "rainy days" when no food may be available. Human catabolic pathways cannot convert fats into proteins. To reiterate, increased protein intake through increased food intake is essential for building muscles.

Second,

Overweight and obese people must avoid molecular roller coasters. Specifically, this includes full attention to the issues of food and mold allergies, glandular and hormonal diseases, and immune disorders.

Third,

Obese people are energy-starved while their fat cells are bloated with oxidized and denatured fats such as trans fatty acids, endoperoxides and cyclic fats. Oxidized fats along with residues of pesticides and preservatives inactivate lipase and other enzymes in the fat cell that regulate fat breakdown and energy generation. The fats in food must be un-oxidized and free of trans fatty acids and toxic cyclic fats. Optimal quantities of reducing and antioxidant vitamins and minerals must be taken to prevent oxidative injury to fats and other nutrients such as amino acids, proteins, carbohydrates and minerals.

Fourth,

The overweight and obese person must do *more* limbic exercises. Limbic (fat-burning) exercises are essential for potentiating fat-burning enzymes. Cortical (sugar-burning) exercises are useful for what nature designed them for: release of quick bursts of energy from sugars for powerful but short-lived muscular movements as in wrestling. See the companion volume *The Ghoraa and Limbic Exercise* for a detailed discussion of this issue.

The overweight person must adopt strategies for ridding his bloated fat cells of toxic fats. Rats fed on supermarket foods rich in oxidized and denatured fats, proteins and sugars as well as foods that contain residues of pesticides and preservatives become obese while rats fed on organically grown foods do not (*Clin Endocrinol Metab* 13:437; 1984). In such rat experiments, the total number of calories in either the supermarket foods or organically grown foods were carefully controlled and matched.

Physicians who practice environmental medicine have clearly documented the harmful effects of pesticides, fungicides, antibiotics, toxic heavy metals and environmental pollutants on human metabolism. I indicated in the preface of this book that, in my view, obesity is caused by catabolic maladaptation that results from eating oxidized, denatured foods and from down-regulation of fat-burning enzymes were the cause of obesity. My hypothesis that the clinical application of the catabolic principle is the primary management strategy for regulating weight evolved after observing patients with environmental illness who always lost some weight as they began to reverse their health disorders.

Increased caloric intake is essential for increasing the muscle mass and enhancing the efficiency of cellular enzymes in muscle cells. In other words, overweight people need more food *to* increase the quantity of their fat-burning enzymes. They also require more activity to enhance the functional efficiency of these enzymes. The fat-burning *thermostat* of the body is up-regulated. *Up-regulation of fat breakdown must be closely balanced with down-regulation of muscle breakdown.*

NUTRIENT INTAKE AND STORED ENERGY

A healthy, lean, energetic person has about 140,000 kcal of energy stored in the form of body fat. In a purely arithmetic sense, with this much stored energy a person can walk for over 400 miles without requiring more food. The energy stored in the form of proteins generally is one-sixth the amount stored as fat (24,000 kcal sufficient to let a person walk about 70 miles). By sharp contrast, the energy stored as glycogen (the main storage form of carbohydrates or sugars) in the muscles, liver, kidney and other tissues is about 800 kcal (barely enough to sustain a walk of one-fourth of a mile).

It follows from the above that the total amount of energy stored in the body as glycogen approximately equals the amount of carbohydrates consumed daily with average meals (200 grams or 800 kcal). Studies have revealed that changes in carbohydrate balance (amount of sugars taken in with food versus amount of sugars utilized for energy) influence the changes in carbohydrate intake on the following day. Predictably, this does not hold for fats; daily fat balance has but little effect on the changes in fat intake on the subsequent day.

The energy requirements of different tissues are different. The brain uses up to 400 kcal per day; the abdominal and chest organs up to 1,000 kcal. At rest, muscle and skin tissues of a nonobese person with sedentary habits use 18% to 20% of his caloric intake.

How much fatty acids are used by the muscle tissue for energy generation? This is a critically important issue in our discussion of the catabolic principle. I indicated above that skin and muscle tissues together burn 18% to 20% of the calories in food in individuals with sedentary habits and untrained muscles. The reason for this is that the fat-catabolic enzymes (oxidative enzymes) are at an ebb in these people. This changes dramatically when the person begins a program designed to increase muscle mass and potentiate fat-burning enzymes. Healthy, lean and vigorous persons burn 50% to 60% of the calories used in their metabolic activities in their muscles.

Physical inactivity is associated with high insulin levels in blood and insulin resistance in tissues. Exercise reverses this by lowering blood insulin levels and decreasing tissue resistance to insulin.

The catabolic principle governs the optimization of weight with up-regulation of fat catabolism and down-regulation of muscle catabolism mass by eating more (not less) food and by eating life-span foods rather than aging-oxidant foods. Up-regulation of fat catabolism means increased fat utilization and fat loss. Down-regulation of muscle catabolism means decreased breakdown of muscle and diminished muscle loss. The end result of the application of the catabolic principle is a lean, fat-free body with a higher level of energy.

MOLECULAR PUNISHMENT BY NIGHT

The goal of applying the catabolic principle to achieve reversal of catabolic maladaptation (and weight loss) is not to try to burn the body fat off by exercise or to starve the fat cells into thinness by dieting. Rather, the goal is to increase the catabolic efficiency of the mitochondrial enzymes by using the principles of life span nutrition and limbic exercise. This is an important distinction that I stress several times in this book.

Let us consider what happens when two friends, one thin

and vigorous and the other obese and sluggish, go out for dinner. They eat a lavish meal of rich, creamy potato soup; beefsteak; baked potatoes with butter; rolls; and a rich, layered chocolate cake for dessert. They have some wine with the meal and espresso coffee with sugar at the end. The total number of calories in the meal is 1755. Now they decide to burn these calories by walking. How long do they need to walk to burn as many calories? At the speed of 5 miles per hour, they will need to walk for 3 hours to burn 1755 calories. Are they likely to do so? Most likely not. But let us suppose they do so. What is likely to happen if they did walk for three hours? The probability is that they will stop at some eating place— perhaps on the suggestion of the overweight friend, after the walk and some more food. A slice or two of pizza perhaps. There is even the probability that after walking for three hours, they may want a full meal again. Clearly, it is simply not a feasible strategy to burn off the calories consumed by walking or with some other exercise after each meal.

Now let us consider what might happen if they were return to their homes and go straight to their beds. What would happen to the food in the body of the thin friend? What would be the fate of the food in the body of the obese friend? Would there be a difference? If so, what? These are critical questions if we are to understand the catabolic principle.

In the bodies of both friends, the digestive processes will break down the foods into simple sugars, amino acids and peptides, and fatty acids and glycerol. The mitochondrial energy enzymes will next break these simpler compounds into water and carbon dioxide and release the chemical bond energy for utilization by the body tissues. What do enzymes do with excess energy? They store it as fat for future use. As I mentioned earlier, the energy enzymes are not aware of our grain silos, our refrigerators and our food stamp programs. They do not know when and from where the next meal will come, if it will. What determines how much energy will be used up and how much will be stored as fat? How will it support the thin person? How will it affect the obese friend?

The efficiency of mitochondrial energy enzymes varies with the overall rate of metabolism. The thin friend has a faster metabolic rate and a greater efficiency of metabolic enzymes. The obese friend has a slower metabolism and a lesser efficiency of such enzymes. This basic difference will determine the fate of the same meal in the bodies of two friends. The efficient enzymes of the thin friend will efficiently utilize the energy in the body of the thin friend and will prevent the delivery of an additional load of fats into the fat cells. The inefficient enzymes of the obese friend, by contrast, will not be able to protect him from another assault by fat molecules.

When thin, vigorous people sleep after a heavy meal, their mitochondrial energy enzymes stand guard against fat buildup. When overweight people sleep after a similar meal, their sluggish enzymes fall into a slumber as well; their bodies take molecular punishment by night.

LIFE IS HARMONIC

In *The Cortical Monkey and Healing,* I describe the

essential fluctuating nature of the recovery process in chronic diseases. Drugs suppress symptoms by inactivating or paralyzing enzymes, and their effects are usually recognizable within hours or days. Nondrug management protocols in molecular medicine work in fundamentally different ways. Nutrients, self-regulatory methods and environmental protocols reduce the oxidative stress on our molecular pathways in a slow and sustained fashion. Still, there are periods of molecular overshoot and compensatory slow downs. These factors create a harmonic effect—peaks of remissions are followed by valleys of relapses. A similar pattern of weight loss and weight gain is observed when catabolic maladaptation is reversed with eating *more* foods and *more* exercise.

MUSCLE IS HEAVIER THAN FAT

There is one other similarity between recovery from chronic disease with nondrug therapies and weight loss by reversal of catabolic maladaptation: Both processes are often accompanied by brief initial periods of a negative trend. The symptoms of a chronic illness may be actually aggravated during an initial, albeit brief, period of nondrug therapies. In reversal of catabolic maladaptation, this phenomenon takes the form of an initial weight gain, or at least a period of no weight loss. One explanation for this, of course, is that muscle tissue is heavier than fat tissue, and the exercise done as a part of the total program leads to a desirable and necessary increase in the muscle mass that outpaces the loss in body fat. For this reason, it is useful to measure the girth of the individual at the beginning of the program and monitor it closely so that this initial positive sign is not misinterpreted as a discouraging negative development.

The diagram that follows schematically illustrates the harmonic pattern of weight gain and loss often seen in the clinical application of the catabolic principle. Some of the peaks of weight loss and valleys of weight gain are due to changes in the amount of life span and aging-oxidant foods eaten and exercise done or omitted. Some changes appear to be related to the expected variation with which an individual can be expected to follow the program. Some other factors appear to be biologic in nature, and seem to represent molecular and enzymatic adjustments.

The Catabolic Principle

Weight Loss

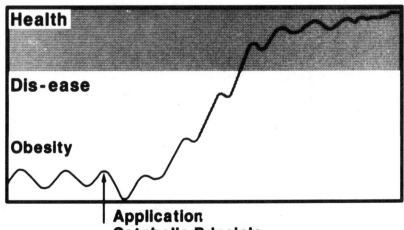

Health

Dis-ease

Obesity

Application
Catabolic Principle

Catabolic Principle Illustrated

The clinical application of catabolic principle for attaining and maintaining the life-span weight is schematically shown in the following two graphs. The first graph shows the data for dynamic changes seen in the body weight of an overweight person who is on a dieting program that reduces the caloric intake in steps. The second graph shows the data for an overweight person on a weight-loss program based on the catabolic principle.

Obesity: A Catabolic Maladaptation

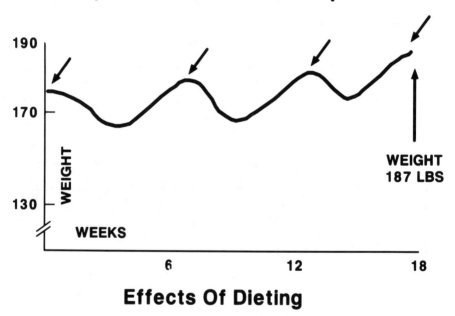

Effects Of Dieting

The above graph shows the effects of dieting on the weight of the patient and the damage done by dieting. With dieting, the individual initially loses weight, mostly by losing body water and body muscle. This gives him a false sense of hope. He does not appreciate that dieting makes him flabby and tired. With muscle loss, and the loss of fat-burning enzymes that always accompanies it, the body's ability to burn fat is further diminished.

The patient in the above figure initially weighed 178 pounds and was on a 1,900 calorie per day diet at the start of a weight-loss program which included dieting. His caloric intake was gradually reduced from 1,900 calories to 1,550. After the initial weight loss of 18 pounds, he gained 22 pounds, at which time his calories were reduced from 1,550 to 1,350. Again he lost weight, only to regain the lost weight and add yet another five pounds. His calories were then reduced from 1,350 to 1,100. Again he lost weight, only to regain his previous weight and add still more pounds, his final weight being 187. With each cycle of reducing his caloric intake, he further lost muscle mass and his ability to catabolize fats.

Veteran dieters will readily recognize this pattern. The weight of an obese person begins to rise again, even though he or she eats less food with dieting. Further attempts to lose weight by eating less food result in a repetition of the whole cycle: less food, more muscle loss, fewer fat-burning enzymes, and still more weight gain even though the obese person is now eating less than he or she was eating during the first round of dieting. With each round of dieting, the problem of obesity worsens.

In the second case history illustrated below, the application of the catabolic principle produced an exact opposite pattern of progressive weight loss as a result of increasing the intake of food. At the start of the program, this person weighed 180 pounds and he was on a punishing diet of 950 calories. (This may surprise some readers but is not very rare among many persons who have been the misfortune of receiving very poor advice.) His ending weight and caloric intake were 141 pounds and 2,100 calories respectively. The key differences between the two case studies resulted from progressive limbic exercises and progressive increments in the caloric intake for the patient on the catabolic principle program. Overweight and obese people who have successfully shed pounds will also see this pattern readily, even though they may not have appreciated the catabolic basis of their positive change.

Obesity: A Catabolic Maladaptation

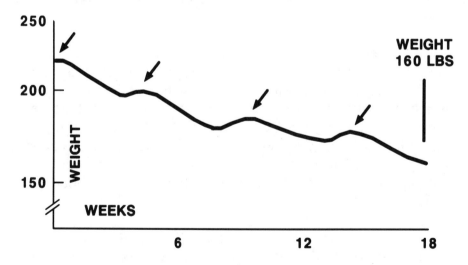

Effects of Applied Catabolic Principle

I indicated earlier that to achieve and maintain life span weight, a person must begin by eating more life span foods and avoiding aging-oxidant foods under close professional supervision. He or she also needs to embarks upon a schedule of progressive limbic exercises. All issues of food and mold allergy, chemical sensitivity, metabolic disorders, glandular insufficiencies, and stress must be addressed. As the individual begins to feel progressively more energetic, he must do limbic exercise (See the companion volume, *The Ghoraa and Limbic Exercise.* I discuss the type and duration of the initial exercise program in this book at length.) As he gains muscle mass (proven with lean body mass analysis), he should increase the duration of limbic exercise. The desired up-regulation of fat-burning enzymes (the increase in the quantity and efficiency of enzymes) follows as a natural consequence of eating more life span foods and doing more limbic exercise.

This should be followed by yet another increase in the amount of foods eaten followed by a corresponding increase in the duration of limbic exercise. At each subsequent step, he or she should eat more life span foods under professional supervision, become more energetic, gain still more muscle and fat-burning enzymes, and lose yet more weight. This cycle needs to be repeated under the close scrutiny of a knowledgeable professional as many times as necessary until the life span weight is attained and maintained without further changes in the quantity of food eaten and limbic exercises done.

An essential aspect of the clinical application of the catabolic principle is this: With time, the body weight stabilizes at an optimal point, and the person learns to prefer life span foods over aging-oxidant foods as well as to balance the quantity of food eaten with the duration of limbic exercise at an intuitive-visceral level. There is then no need to count calories. No need to fret over food choices. No need to check one's weight every day. A person exercises not because it prevents weight gain or lowers LDL cholesterol or raises HDL cholesterol. None of this is relevant anymore.

My own weight fluctuated between 169 and 135 pounds during the time I was experimenting with it and studying the effects of various types of foods and exercise upon it. Now it has been stable at 142 to 144 pounds for the last several years. I do not recall the last time I weighed myself. (One of the editors who read the manuscript of this chapter wrote on the border of this page, "Then how do you know how much you weigh?" The answer: I just *know*. With time a person reaches a state when he becomes free, free of conscious efforts to choose foods, free of struggle to engage in exercise, even free of a need to know.) I do not recall the last time I did eat or didn't eat anything specifically because of weight considerations. I seem to stay at what appears to me to be my optimal weight, naturally and effortlessly. Indeed, weight consciousness is not a part of my day.

****

The butterfly flies down and in
and then it flies up and out.

Chapter 8

Life Span Food Choices and Aging-Oxidant Foods

*Life span nutrition is a philosophy of food
and its relationship to the human condition.*

Life span nutrition means respecting food so it can respect us.

Life span nutrition is not a "diet". It is *knowing* what we eat. It is knowing how food affects us after we eat it — after some minutes, after some hours, after some days, after some months and after some years. It is knowing how the food we eat affects our *life span.*

Life span nutrition is neither euphoria of eating nor denial of dieting.

Life span nutrition is not about martyrdom before we eat or guilt after it. It is not about calorie counting. It is not about dieting. It is not about starving-gorging-starving cycles.

Life span nutrition is not about "low sugar," "high protein," "low fat" or "mega vitamin" regimens.

Life span nutrition is not about losing weight, though loss of excess weight occurs as a natural consequence of *knowing* the relationship between food and life.

Life span nutrition is a lifelong interest. It is about feeling better, looking better, and living better. It is *about a slow and sustained* change in the way we think about food, feel about it, and are nourished by it.

My philosophy of life span nutrition evolved over several years of clinical work with persons with severe immune and degenerative disorders. It represents a blending of the enormous intuitive wisdom of the ancients in matters of food and my concept that spontaneity of oxidation in nature is the essential cause of the aging process, and by natural extension of premature aging, dis-ease, disease and death. In the preface of this volume, I defined the term life span foods as foods that promote optimal health for the full life span of an individual. I define aging-oxidant foods as foods that cause accelerated (premature) aging.

Foods, like people, have their life spans. Foods, like people, can either live out their normal life spans or they can be subjected to premature aging. Just as we humans suffer from degenerative diseases when we abuse our bodies (or when viruses and bacteria abuse us), our foods suffer from degenerations when they are abused by toxic fumigants, pesticides and chemical preservatives. It is one of the great ironies of our time that we abuse our foods by using "preservative." Foods may be eaten while they are *young* and healthful or when they have grown old and *degenerated*.

The subject of human life span cannot be separated from the subject of life span of our foods. I present below a brief outline of my view of the essential energy and biochemical basis of the aging process in man and accelerated (premature) aging caused by stressors in our internal and external environment. It seems to me that these simplified but scientifically sound concepts are necessary for understanding the relationship between food and the human condition. I strongly urge the reader without a biology background to read the next few pages carefully, and if necessary, reread and reread them until he is completely familiar with the basic scientific knowledge that forms the basics of life span nutrition described in this chapter. Following a brief discussion of these scientific principles, I cite specific examples of living foods and dead foods to illustrate these principles in a practical sense.

I refer the professional reader to my monograph *Intravenous Nutrient Protocols in Molecular Medicine* for an in-depth discussion of the molecular dynamics of plasma membranes, oxidative enzymatic pathways, and the molecular counterbalance provided by life span molecules.

I want to prove --- that the boundaries set by the Gods are not unbreakable.

Gilgamesh 5000 B.C.

Each living thing must one day die. If it had not been so for one single life form, that life form would have lived for ever and would have crowded out all other forms of life from the planet Earth.

If one species of fish had lived for ever, it would have filled up all the oceans, seas, rivers and lakes on our planet. There would have been no room for any other species of fish. Or for any other form of life in the water, any mollusk, any crab, any algae. If one single species of plant or animal on earth were to be exempt from nature's "law of death", that plant or animal would have packed every inch of the land. There would have been no room for a new twig, a new bloom, a new plant, a new insect or a new baby. I wonder if Gilgamesh knew this.

Life must be preceded by death. Life, it seems to me, can be understood only through death.

How did nature design this death-life-death cycle? Nature is master planner. It is an ingenious designer. It has its own economy. It rarely errs. It is self-correcting.

Recycling life is one of nature's master stroke.

Oxidation is nature's grand design for assuring that no life form lives for ever. Nature made oxidation a spontaneous process. It requires no expenditure of energy. It needs no external cues or outside programming. In scientific jargon, oxidation is defined as *loss* of electron by atoms and molecules. A molecule is a group of atoms bonded together. Electrons are the tiniest packets of energy. When atoms and molecules lose electrons, they lose energy. In oxidation, high-energy atoms and molecules are changed into lower-energy level atoms and molecules. *This is the essence of the phenomenon of aging.*

In the mid-sixties, Bjorksten and Harmon put forth their theories of protein cross-linking and free radical injury respectively as the basic mechanisms of the aging process. Healthy threadlike protein molecules normally occur in different sizes. Individual molecules are bent and turned and twisted into many different shapes. Yet, they fight hard to preserve their individuality. The term cross-linking means these molecules are torn apart and when the ends unite, they get tangled with each other and form crooked protein molecules. Cross-linked molecules are two molecules wrapped around each other in such a way that neither can function normally. What molecular events cause protein cross-linking? Oxidative injury. It is the oxidant molecules that tear apart the health protein molecules and lead to tangling and cross-linking of these molecules.

How does free radical injury begin? With oxidative injury. Free radicals are highly unstable, extremely reactive atoms or molecules that form when oxidant molecules injure other molecules. Aging of human tissues and molecules cannot take place by free radical injury unless these radicals are first produced as a result of oxidation. It follows that *spontaneity of oxidation* in human tissues, and oxidative molecular injury that results, may be regarded as the *true* nature of the aging process in man. Tissue capacity for anti-oxidant generation (production of life span molecules to control the aging-oxidant molecules and related molecules called oxyradicals) is determined by certain genetic and acquired factors. Life span molecules so produced provide the essential molecular counterbalance to spontaneous oxidation. I draw the evidence for this viewpoint from a large body of clinical and experimental data.

THE AGING-OXIDANT MOLECULES AOM

During the early period of the development of my theory of life span and aging-oxidant foods, I often wondered if these terms were suitable for communicating my ideas of health and fitness to my patients. I started using these terms tentatively in my seminars on nutrition for the life span. I soon discovered that patients without any biology background at all could understand these terms, and the essential ideas behind their use, easily and effortlessly. Indeed, people found the simplified concept of molecular aging, disease and death described with these two terms a useful framework for understanding nutrition. Below is a brief explanation of these terms.

The AOMs exist to assure that no life forms lives forever. These molecules are present in each flower, each plant, each animal and each person. These are powerful molecules, fully capable of instantaneously burning all tissues. The AOMs can be divided into two broad categories: the internal metabolic AOMs and the external synthetic and natural toxic AOMS. The examples of the first category include aging-oxidant metabolic enzymes, minerals, proteins, fats and stress molecules. The external AOMs include industrial pollutants, petrochemicals, synthetic household chemicals, antibiotics, pesticides and herbicides. Radioactivity, ultraviolet waves and other forms of radiation do not come under the strict definition of AOMs, but readily generate AOMs by acting upon various atoms and molecules.

THE LIFE SPAN MOLECULES *LSM*

Life span molecules are molecules that provide a counterbalance to aging-oxidant molecules. These molecules exist to assure that the aging-oxidant molecules do not cause instant combustion of all living forms. As each flower, each plant, each animal and each person is made up of AOMs, so it is made up of LSMs. LSMs exist to provide a counterbalance to AOMs. These molecules "neutralize" AOMs and prevent unwanted tissue damage. It is their responsibility is to assure that each life form gets the opportunity to live out its normal life span in health, and with vigor and vitality. Examples of such molecules are vitamins, essential fatty acids, essential amino acids, essential minerals, and other antioxidants.

ENZYMES:
LIFE FORCE OF FOODS IN NATURE.

Enzymes are molecules that separate living organisms from nonliving objects. Enzymes are catalysts in biologic reactions; these molecules facilitate reactions between other molecules but in general are not used up in those reactions. They "make things happen" between other molecules. Indeed, enzymes *are* life.

Foods in nature are living things. Enzymes are what gives foods in Nature their life. Indeed, enzymes *are* the life in foods. If this is true, why is the subject of enzymes in human nutrition almost completely neglected by our nutrition experts? The answer to this question has something to do with the limitations of the available methods of scientific inquiry. The prevailing research models do not allow us to fully understand the *quality* of life in enzymes.

Man has not been able to fully understand what life is. His science has not been able to define what life is. Since the time modern man walked out of the Rift Valley in central Africa (or so paleohistorians want us to believe), he has searched for the true meaning of what life is and has failed consistently. In frustration, he has expressed the essential *nature* of life as *vital force, life force, energy force,* or simply *vitality.* Indeed, the poet and the philosopher have always been closer to describing the *quality* of life than the scientist.

Returning to the subject of enzymes in foods, it is essential to recognize that what brings proteins, fats, carbohydrates and minerals to life is enzymes. Without enzymes, these substances would be nothing but lifeless masses of molecules. Casimer Funk recognized the *vital* importance of some substances to health, and his "substances" were called *vitamins.* Most vitamins *are* enzymes. Those that do not meet the biochemical characteristics to be considered enzymes, primarily act to facilitate enzymes.

To understand what enzymes are and how they function, let us consider the example of automobile wheels moving on a road surface. When the road surface is dry, the wheels "hug" the road and the driver is in easy command of his vehicle. When it rains and the road surface is wet, the wheels do not hug the road as well. The driver senses this change and slows down to improve his control over his vehicle. During a freezing rain, ice prevents the wheels from hugging the road surface, and the vehicle slides uncontrollably. If the driver does not slow down his vehicle to a crawl or a stop, he may find himself in a ditch by the roadside. How does this happen? The answer: The water reduces the friction between the tire and the road (facilitates the "reaction" between the two). The play of the tire on the road surface is looser and freer, and it loses its grip on the road surface. The driver senses some difficulty of control. When water freezes, the smooth surface of the ice almost completely eliminates friction between the tire and the road surface. The driver cannot cope with such rapid play of the tire on the road and unless he slows down.

In the above analogy, water acts as an enzyme. It is not used up but simply facilitates the movement ("reaction") between the surfaces of the tire and the road (reduces friction between the two in common language). So enzymes are life molecules that *make things happen in living organisms.*

THE LIFE SPAN AND AGING-OXIDANT ENZYMES

Historically, the enzymes in the human body have been classified into two broad groups: the digestive enzymes and the metabolic enzymes. This was a valid classification. I say it *was* because this classification was developed and taught before we realized the devastating impact of synthetic chemicals and toxic metals on human biology.

From an ecologic viewpoint, it seems to me, it is useful to separate enzymes into *life span enzymes* (enzymes that support life span molecules) and *aging-oxidant enzymes* (enzymes that facilitate the destructive-oxidative function of aging-oxidant molecules). Just as nature designed some molecules to assure that no life form lives forever, it designed some enzymes for the same reason. Similarly, life span enzymes were designed to sustain the living organisms for their life span.

ENZYME BANK FOR LIFE

Each living organism is blessed by nature with a lifetime complement of enzymes, an *enzyme bank* so to speak. Living tissues have a capacity for producing enzymes, but this capacity is clearly limited. We can be prudent with this bank and live well for our life span, or we can be frivolous and waste this finite life resource, age prematurely, and get weak and ill. How can we be prudent with our enzyme bank account? The same way we can be prudent with our regular bank account: by spending it with care and with love for our enzymes.

The principal threat to life on planet Earth is the destruction of its life span enzymes.

If life on our planet is to survive in more or less the same form as we see it today, we will have to think differently about enzymes, the enzymes in our food chain, the enzymes in our tissues, and the enzymes of other living things around us.

We rigorously and systematically destroy enzymes in our food with food-processing technology and denature (cook) them by our high-temperature cooking. Fresh vegetables and fruits are exceptions to this only when they are not laced with pesticides or wrapped with chemical fumigants. Our fruit industry "polishes" as many fruits as it can to make them look pretty, and in the process embeds deeply into their skin toxic designer killer molecules.

Most of the environmental pollutants are poisons for life span enzymes. But this is not where the tragedy of systematic destruction of life span enzymes ends. Many of these enzymes are damaged in such a way that they become instruments of molecular destruction. Many environmental toxins and most drugs convert life span enzymes into aging-oxidant enzymes.

Rarely do we recognize that what poisons insect enzyme also poisons food and human enzymes. Almost all commonly used pesticides (organophosphate and chlorinated compounds) kill insects by poisoning their enzymes, called choline esterases. What we rarely recognize is that most of the insect choline estrases are identical to human choline estrases. What kills the bugs also kills us. If that is true, it may be asked, why don't people also die?

Insects die quickly because there is so little of them to be killed by pesticides. People die slowly because there is so much of them to be killed.

Certain enzymes in our body serve the specific function

of detoxifying synthetic and natural chemicals that gain entry into our bodies. One such group of enzymes is called mixed function oxidase system. In a healthy child, these enzymes function as life span enzymes and neutralize or detoxify drugs and other synthetic molecules. When a child is put on barbiturates and other drugs for long periods of time, these enzymes gear up to handle the drug overload. In scientific jargon, this phenomenon is called enzyme induction and refers to formation of excessive quantities of enzymes which now begin to destroy an individual's own molecules (auto-enzymity?), much like the induced immune system begins to destroy a person's own cells and organs in autoimmune disorders. Another system of enzymes in the body is called cytochrome P 450 system. This system is also designed to detoxify foreign chemicals. Many drugs inactivate these enzyme systems, and such destructive potential of many commonly used drugs, such as Tagamet used for stomach ulcer, is rarely recognized. Failure of this enzyme system has been documented to cause serious chemical toxicity with unrelenting immune injury and chronic illness.

FOOD COMPOSITION AND ENZYME SHIFTS

The subject of digestive enzymes in fresh, uncooked, unprocessed foods is an essential but poorly understood aspect of human nutrition.

Cats and dogs in the wild are carnivorous, and their

saliva contains little if any amylase enzymes for digesting carbohydrates. By contrast, the saliva of domesticated cats and dogs fed high-carbohydrate, high-sugar foods contains large quantities of amylases and other digestive enzymes. How does this happen? The answer is simple: Enzymes in living organisms actively respond to the food they eat. In *The Cortical Monkey and Healing,* I wrote:

Biology is forever changing; we change one thing in one way, we change everything in some way.

Wild cats and dogs eat unprocessed food that contains its own digestive enzymes. By allowing the enzymes in their food to partly digest their foods, they in effect conserve their own digestive enzymes. Similarly, the weight and size of rat pancreas varies with the nature of food eaten by rats. A wild rat has a smaller pancreas than a laboratory rat who is fed a heat-processed, enzyme-free diet. (Edward Howell, *Enzyme Nutrition,* Avery Publishing, 1985).

LOST WISDOM, LOST ENZYMES

A tragic casualty of our infatuation with the "science" of nutrition is the lost wisdom of the ancients. How could we so arrogantly dismiss their wisdom as "old wives tales"? (Show me a person who snubs others with this phrase, and I will show you a person who has been robbed of his capacity for quiet reflection on the nature of things). I consider the wisdom of the ancients in matters of human nutrition the bedrock of all strategies for sound nutrition for the life span. *True* bits of nutrition science (structure and function of nutrient molecules) must be woven into the texture of the cumulative wisdom of mankind vis-a-vis the relationship between food and the human condition.

The ancient knew of many ways to enhance the nutritional value of their foods. Soybean makes for an illuminating case study.

Soybean is an excellent sources of minerals such as magnesium, calcium, molybdenum and others. It has a rich content of some "life span oils". In our recent research studies with positively and negatively charged soybean glycolipids, my co-researcher and nutrition scientist, Gary Viole, and I have observed some extraordinary benefits of these natural products for patients with irritable bowel syndrome, ulcerative colitis, Crohn's colitis and related chronic inflammatory bowel disorders. And, of course, soybean has high-quality proteins. It comes close to being a perfect food. But there is something more to it.

Soybean is a seed. Like all other seeds, it is rich in enzyme inhibitors. Here is another master stroke of nature. Seeds are nature's tiny parcels of future life. They must be preserved. They must be protected not only from the vicissitudes of their environments but also from the enzymes within them. These enzymes are designed to cause autodigestion and breakdown (the law of death in nature). So Nature gave them outer shells and inner molecular safety in the form of enzyme inhibitors.

The ancients seemed to have intuitively known about these nutritional aspects of soybean, even though little comes down to us about their insights in these matters in a well-documented form. Why else would they hold it in such high esteem? Also they seemed to have recognized the problem of enzyme inhibitors in soybean. Why else would they be so inventive about the matters of antidigestive (enzyme inhibitors) aspects of soybean? Why else would they prepare soybean dishes in so many ways with the specific result of neutralizing and predigesting it?

The ancient Chinese mastered the art of neutralizing enzyme inhibitors and predigesting soybean with several fungus enzymes, mostly from Aspergillus species. They literally "cooked" their soybean with fungus enzymes. There is, however, a critical difference between cooking soybean (and other foods) with heat and cooking them with fungus enzymes: Cooking with heat destroys life enzymes while cooking with enzymes increases the life enzyme content of foods.

Tofu kan, yuba, and *tofu p'i* were the names they gave to their soybean dishes prepared for the specific purpose of increasing its digestibility by adding to it life enzymes of fungi (and for conserving their own digestive enzymes). They enhanced its nutritional value and at the same time spared their own enzymes. They were prudent about their own life enzyme banks. The Chinese also used soybean curd to prepare another dish called *kabitofu.* The people in Philippines called their favorite partially digested soybean dish *toya.* The well-known *tofu* is a "cheese" made up of partially digested soybean. *Natto* is the name given to a similar product. For many centuries, people of Java treated their soybean with enzymes and named their dish *tempeh.*

The Japanese were not to be left behind in this competition for saving their life span enzymes. They perfected *miso,* a fermented soybean food used as porridge at breakfast. The Japanese also experimented with other grains and made *miso* with barley and rice.

The principle of predigesting foods with natural substances to enhance its nutritional value (conserving the life enzyme bank account in our jargon) is not the sole cultural heritage of people of the Far East. Yogurt was the prime predigested food of ancient India. Cheeses were the predigested foods of early Europeans. They prepared their cheese to enhance its nutritional value and for specific taste goals by treating it with specific bacterial enzymes.

Predigestion of food is an old discovery of man. In almost all of his cultures and in all eras of his history, man has used the principle of predigesting his food by borrowing digestive enzymes from other forms of life. Today we find some of its early applications repulsive, even barbaric. Jivaros Indians of the Amazon River basin prepared *nijimanche* by thoroughly chewing the yucca bark and spitting it into large jars where its digestion by amylase enzymes of the saliva continued for hours. They treasured this drink for its nutritional value. We do not need to adopt their specific methods, but we must recognize the relevance of their insights into the matters of food digestion to our health today. Their food "packaging" appears repugnant to our delicate taste and sensibility today. Little do we realize that they, in their barbaric primitiveness, were much truer to their food than we who hide toxic foods in elegant packaging.

Soybean is the current favorite for preparing predigested foods among people interested in their food and health. It is unfortunate that our food industry does not see the intuitive wisdom of the ancient and build upon it for healthier foods with abundant life span enzymes. The ancient perfected the art of preparing healthful predigested foods and drinks. We can both adopt and adapt their methods. Enzyme foods and beverages, as Edward Howell and others have suggested, can be prepared in many aesthetically pleasing ways.

The Basic Equation of Life

The balance between the AOMs and LSMs is the basic equation of life. In scientific jargon, it is called *redox reaction*. The redox equilibrium (or potential as it is sometimes called) determines the health and life of foods as it determines the health and life of people, animals and plants.

Human biology is an ever-changing kaleidoscope of molecular mosaics. AOMs and LSMs are in dynamic equilibrium at all times. Health and disease — at energy, electron and molecular levels — can be defined as the states created by the impact of AOMs and LSMs on an individual's genetic makeup. Health, in this light, may be seen as a dynamic state in which the LSMs have the upper hand, and preserve the structural and functional integrity of cells and tissues. Disease, by contrast, is a state in which AOMs overwhelm the LSMs and cause dis-ease and disease.

I call the clinical practice of medicine founded on this basic equation of life molecular medicine, a medicine of future that seeks to reverse the basic cause of disease rather than simply suppress the symptoms with drugs. In acute illness, we need drugs or surgical scalpels. In chronic disease, nondrug treatment protocols of nutritional medicine, environmental medicine, medicine of self-regulation and fitness offer clearly superior long-term results.

How Do We Age?

① Human frames age when their body organ age.
② Human body organs age when their tissues age.
③ Human tissues age when their cells age.
④ Human cells age when their molecules age.
⑤ Human molecules age when they lose their plasticity.

How do molecules lose their plasticity? By oxidative injury. Oxidative molecular damage, then, is the *true* nature of molecular aging.

Molecular Duality of Oxygen

Oxygen builds molecules.
Oxygen lacerates, mutilates and destroys molecules.
Oxygen sustains life.
Oxygen terminates life.

How does a log of wood burn to give us fire for cooking our meals? It requires oxygen to burn. It burns with oxygen. In the process of burning, the log yields its energy and turns into ashes. Oxygen serves our body tissues in exactly the same way. Food materials yield their chemical bond energy as they are burned by oxygen. We use this energy both for the processes of life and for building up our body stores of energy for periods when foods may not be available to us.

How do our enzymes build the molecules for the

structure and function of the various tissues in our body? With oxygen. Oxygen and enzymes do not seem to care about our notions of eating or dieting. I am convinced our metabolic enzymes still do not know about our refrigerators, our food stamp programs, and about our grain silos. The enzymes maintain a high level of preparedness for a famine even when we indulge in heavy eating. They do not know where our next meal might come from or whether or not there will be a next meal.

Oxygen is a molecular Dr. Jekyll and Mr. Hyde.

Human nutrition cannot be understood without understanding the duality of oxygen. This is the master stroke of nature. What brings forth life also terminates life.

Threat of extinction by accelerated oxidative injury — an insight from nature.

Mankind faces a clear threat of extinction today. We have enormously increased the aging-oxidant stress on our tissues. The molecules of stress of modern life (adrenaline and its cousin molecules) are powerful oxyradicals. Toxic metals leached from the soil by acid rain and poured into our cells with drinking water are powerful oxyradicals. Pesticides and fungicides are *designer* killer molecules because they are oxyradicals. Antibiotics kill bad germs as well as good germs. They act as powerful oxyradicals. Industrial pollutants are powerful oxyradicals. Indeed, we live beneath an avalanche of synthetic chemicals that act as oxyradicals, directly or indirectly.

Proto-eukaryotes were tiny single-cell ancestors of our cells. Early proto-eukaryotes of planet Earth were sustained by a largely oxygen-free atmosphere. Their survival was threatened as blue algae acquired photosynthetic activity (ability to convert solar energy into chemical bond energy) and began to release large quantities of oxygen into the atmosphere. Pro-karyotes are another type of single-cell organisms that can utilize oxygen. In the late 1960s, Lynn Margulis, Ph.D., of Massachusetts, proposed that mitochondria and certain other cellular organelles evolved from certain oxygen-utilizing prokaryotes that migrated into the bodies of proto-eukaryotes. Mitochondria, I described earlier in the chapter On the Nature of Obesity, are tiny sausage-shaped structures within the cells that contain energy generating oxidative enzymes of cells.

In this symbiotic relationship between the proto-karyotes and pro-karyotes, the former provided prokaryotes a safe environment. The prokaryotes, in turn, saved proto-karyotes from oxygen toxicity. The Margulis theory was validated by subsequent studies. Can man evolve new molecular defenses rapidly enough to protect him from extinction by oxyradicals? The answer: Molecular evolution occurs over a period of millions of years. Molecular evolution cannot be served up as a take-out meal. We need a new and a different view of our molecules, of our tissues, of the life around us, of our planet Earth.

What are the clinical implications of this viewpoint of aging in man? Oxygen is a molecular Dr. Jekyll and Mr. Hyde. Life-sustaining aspects of oxygen are well understood in clinical medicine. Life-terminating capability of oxygen is generally ignored. Man today faces extinction by accelerated oxidative molecular damage much like proto-eukaryotes did during an earlier era. This accelerated oxidative stress is caused by the impact upon his genetic makeup of an enormous overload of aging-oxidant molecules on his internal and external environment. What are the best strategies for health promotion and reversal of chronic immunologic and degenerative disorders? These are the strategies that address *all* aspects of accelerated oxidative molecular injury. These are the clinical management protocols of nutritional medicine, environmental medicine, medicine of self-regulation and medicine of fitness. Integrated applications of such management protocols is the clinical practice of molecular medicine.

What is the language of molecular injury?

Oxidation.

****

What is the language of molecular recovery?

Reduction.

****

What is the language of molecular aging?

Oxidative molecular injury.

****

What is the true nature of the aging process?

Spontaneity of oxidation in nature.

Life Spans of Foods

Foods, like people and plants, have their life spans. The life span of food items is determined by the balance between their AOMs and LSMs, just as it occurs in people and plants. Food items contain sugars, proteins and fats for their *own* metabolism. We consume foods as components of our food chain. Foods also contain enzymes, vitamins and minerals, again to preserve their own life span and health. Food molecules get injured and get *sick* the same way people do.

Electron transfer, free radical production and destruction, enzymatic detoxification, and metabolic breakdown occur in food molecules in ways that are very similar to those in the human body. Furthermore, the life span of food items is preserved by mechanisms that are almost identical to ours.

Is the concept of life span of foods relevant to life span nutrition? Are the life span mechanisms of foods of concern to us?

FOODS SPOIL BY OXIDATIVE DAMAGE

Foods spoil due to molecular oxidative stress. Let us consider some examples.

An apple falls on the kitchen floor and is bruised. Hours later, the pulp under the bruised area of skin becomes softened and turns color. How does it happen? Apple skin contains bioflavinoids that serve as apple antioxidants and prevent oxygen in the air from causing oxidative injury to the skin and the pulp beneath it. When the skin of the apple is bruised with a fall, it develops tiny microscopic cracks. Oxygen in the air gains entry into the substance of the apple skin and apple pulp and activates the aging-oxidative enzymes contained in the cells there. Unlike human tissues, the apple "tissues" do not have much capacity for generating life span molecules. The expected result: The apple skin and pulp are oxidatively damaged, turn brown and spoil.

Lettuce is rich in vitamin C, a strong life span molecule. Vitamin C, along with other plant LSMs contained in lettuce, prevents oxidative browning and spoiling of lettuce. When lettuce is finely chopped and exposed to oxygen in the air, it suffers the same oxidative damage as that of a bruised apple. Within several minutes, sixty to eighty percent of vitamin C and other LSMs contained in lettuce get oxidized. Within some hours, lettuce is oxidatively damaged, turns brown and spoils.

Fresh flaxseed oil is pale gold and has a pleasant flavor. Linseed seeds are rich in omega-6 oils that serve the seed as its LSMs. The seeds of the flaxseed plant carry omega-6 oils to preserve their own health and to use them as a source of energy. Omega-6 oils are high-energy molecules. Animals and people eat plant foods like flaxseed seeds and draw their supply of these essential fatty acids. Omega-6 oils stabilize cell plasma membranes and keep these membranes fluid and functional. In nature, high-energy molecules show a natural tendency to lose their electrons and "decay" into lower-level energy molecules.

Fortunately, this is a slow process. The seeds of the flaxseed and other plants use their LSMs to keep their omega-6 oils in their native high-energy state for long periods of time. But the seed LSMs are helpless against the mutilation of their molecules by our food processing technologies.

The primary commitment of the food industry is to its bottom line. It sees profits in longer shelf lives of its foods. So what does it do? It processes the flaxseed oil to increase its shelf-life, and in doing so changes high-energy state oils into low-energy state molecules. The "clear" oils so produced do not spoil for long periods because there is not much left in them to spoil. And that's not all. During processing, the food oils get oxidized, partially denatured, and contaminated with variable quantities of toxic cyclic products of fat breakdown. Flaxseed oil is oxidatively damaged and spoils. The food technology starts with a life span oil and turns it into an aging-oxidant oil.

Flaxseed oil should be purchased only if packaged in dark brown or black bottles (to reduce the rate of oxidation by light energy), 1000 to 3000 units of vitamin E should be added to slow down the natural rate of oxidation, and the bottle should be refrigerated. Needless to say, flaxseed oil should be taken cold, as a salad dressing ingredient or simply as food supplement.

In the above three examples, the life span of foods is shortened and the nutritive value of food markedly diminished by premature oxidative damage of foods.

Injured foods injure healthy tissues.

This is self-evident but seldom fully appreciated. The four *whites* (white flour, white sugar, white rice and white oil) are prime examples of how we injure our foods. These are also prime examples of how injured foods injure our tissues. Our tissues can be expected to prematurely age, and they do, when we sustain them with prematurely aged foods.

LIFE SPAN MOLECULES SUSTAIN HUMAN LIFE SPAN

Life-span molecules sustain the species life span in two important ways. First, life-span foods preserve the structural integrity of human cells. Second, life-span foods preserve the functional capacity of the cells. I cite two of my recent research studies to illustrate these phenomena. In those studies, I examined the effects of vitamin C on the structure of the cell membrane of red blood cells and on the function of the plasma membrane of platelets, the smallest of all blood corpuscles. The stickiness of blood platelets plays a central role in the causation of heart attack, stroke and other vascular problems.

Ascorbic acid reverses abnormal erythrocyte morphology in chronic fatigue syndrome.

Ali, M. Am J Clin Pathol 94:515, 1990

In the preceding study, I examined the membrane of red blood cells of patients with allergy caused by IgE-type antibodies and who suffered from chronic persistent fatigue. I used a high-resolution microscope that enlarges the red corpuscles of blood over 11,000 times. I observed that up to 50% of all red cells showed marked deformities of the red blood cell membrane. Some of these cells had wrinkled membranes, others showed sharp angulations, and yet others bore thornlike projections on their surfaces. It was evident to me that blood cells with such deformities could not flow smoothly within the blood capillaries. It seems to me that this is one of the causes of muscle and skin pains, aches and numbness which patients with chronic fatigue often suffer. In the second part of that study, I examined the effects of vitamin C on the deformed cell membranes. Following an intravenous infusion of 15 grams of ascorbic acid (vitamin C), the regular structure of the red blood cell membrane was restored in more than half of the cells showing abnormalities. The study demonstrates the efficacy of vitamin C in restoring the structural integrity of the erythrocyte membrane, and by implication, the membranes of cells of other tissues. Ascorbic acid appears to restore the normal erythrocyte morphology by reducing the oxidant stress imposed upon it by allergic triggers and other factors.

Ascorbic acid prevents platelet aggregations by norepinephrine, collagen, ADP and ristocetin.

Ali, M. Am J Clin Pathol 95:281, 1991

In the second study, I investigated the effects of ascorbic

acid on the function of platelet plasma membranes. In my laboratory, I caused the blood platelets to become sticky and form platelet clots (platelet aggregates) by exposing them to the oxidative stress of adrenaline and three other substances identified in the title of the paper cited above. I fully expected that vitamin C would protect the platelets from the oxidative stress of adrenaline and prevent abnormal stickiness. That is indeed what I observed. What I had not expected, and it turned out to be a far more important observation, was that vitamin C would cause the breakup of formed platelet clots (dissociation of formed platelet aggregates). These data suggest strongly that ascorbic acid may be of great value in the prevention of heart attack, stroke and other vascular problems that begin with formation of platelet clots. I believe further studies will validate my observations, and vitamin C will be accepted as a far superior food factor for prevention of these diseases than aspirin, which is presently used for this purpose. Aspirin, as is well known, causes stomach bleeding, tiny ulcers in the stomach lining and in many cases leads to abnormal patterns of bleeding.

VITAMIN C: A GUARDIAN ANGEL MOLECULE FOR THE HEART

Recently, Linus Pauling and Matthias Rath proposed another protective role of vitamin C in the prevention of arteriosclerosis which leads to heart attacks and strokes. They hypothesized that lipoprotein (a) is a surrogate for ascorbate (*Proc. Natl. Acad. Sci* 87:6204; 1990). The evidence they marshaled to support their hypothesis includes the following: 1) Lipoprotein is generally found in the blood of primates and guinea pig, which have lost the ability to synthesize vitamin C; 2) lipoprotein shares with vitamin C the properties of facilitating wound healing and preventing lipid peroxidation; 3) High lipoprotein levels in blood are associated with heart disease; and 4) The incidence of heart disease is decreased by elevated levels of vitamin C.

A large number of studies show the many ways vitamin C prevents oxidative injury to other life molecules and prevents tissue injury and diseases. Two of my own studies briefly described above show some of the other ways vitamin C acts as the guardian angel molecule for the heart. I discussed this subject at length in a recent review article which appeared in the winter 1991 issue of *The Environmental Physician* published by the American Academy of Environmental Medicine. I include below some brief comments.

VITAMIN C: A PREMIUM LIFE SPAN MOLECULE.

Vitamin C is an excellent life span molecule. It is a molecule of small size, a close cousin of the glucose molecule from which it is derived in animals. We human beings cannot make this vitamin from glucose molecules because we do not have an enzyme necessary for this. It has been estimated that we humans lost the enzyme (glucunolactone oxidase) over 50 million years ago. Vitamin C is water soluble, is freely cleared through the kidneys and the bowel. It has no known toxicity. It is a premium water-soluble anti-oxidant molecule in the blood (Proc Nat Acad Sci 86:6377;1989). It is essential for the function of several enzymes including some that are necessary for the synthesis of stress molecules in the adrenal gland and the metabolism of cholesterol. Finally and fortunately, no drug company has a patent on it and so it is quite inexpensive.

VITAMIN C IS AN ORPHAN DRUG

I have often thought how different things would have been if a drug company had owned a patent protecting its sale of vitamin C. I have no doubt in my mind that such a patent would have been the greatest blockbuster of all time, an unparalleled gold mine of a patent. I have also wondered how different things would have been in the area of "continuing medical education" for physicians in the hospitals. More lectures on the clinical benefits of this life-span molecule would have been given by doctors (paid by the drug company holding the patent) in our hospitals than for any other drug. The reason for this is simple. The drug researchers would have figured out that vitamin C, a powerful life span molecule, is likely to benefit many clinical disorders, just as physicians in nutritional medicine have found out. The difference is that when drug companies discover something, they spend millions of dollars to disseminate such information for marketing their drugs. When physician-nutritionists discover something of value about vitamin C, there is no money available for spreading this information. So it is that vitamin C remains an orphan drug.

A Balanced Diet: What Is It?

I have been a student of human biology for about 35 years and of human nutrition for about 15 years. I must admit I do not know what a "balanced diet" is.

Next time you meet a nutrition "expert," ask him what he considers a balanced diet. His answer is likely to be this: It is a diet composed of all four major food groups — of dairy, meat, cereal, and fruits and vegetables; it has 50 to 60% of its calories in carbohydrates, 20 to 25% in proteins, and 20 to 25 % in fats; and it contains 60 mg of vitamin C, 1 mg of thiamine and RDA amounts of other vitamins and minerals. If he is very "knowledgeable," he might add that the fats should be one part saturated, one part monosaturated, and one part polyunsaturated.

A sad, sad state of affairs. These nutrition experts are blissfully ignorant of almost all critical nutritional issues we face today. They know nothing (or act as if they don't) about the issues of molecular roller coasters caused by supermarket foods, food incompatibilities, abnormal bowel responses to foods, allergy to molds included in food items, toxic fats, denatured proteins, agricultural fumigants that coat our vegetables, pesticides and fungicides that cover our fruits, the toxic heavy metals that poison our foods, environmental pollutants that contaminate our water, and the industrial toxins that poison our air. Our nutrition experts do not seem to understand much about the molecular consequences of disrupted bowel ecology.

I discuss the scientific aspects of the full impact of food and environmental toxicants upon our immune system and molecular defense systems in my monograph *The Molecular and Immunologic Basis of Environmental Illness* published by the American Academy of Environmental Medicine.

Here is simple test to distinguish between the "experts" of worthless knowledge of nutrition and practitioners of nutritional medicine: If a physician, a nutritionist, or some other health professional talks about RDA values, know that he cannot help you much. He is not even close to the real problems in nutrition.

Here is second simple test: Ask the professional if he has ever reversed any chronic diseases with nutritional protocol. If his answer is no, he is obviously not your man. Some of my physician-colleagues might snicker at this and say,"Of course, I treat anemia with iron and pernicious anemia with vitamin B_{12}. I am sorry, but that, as the expression goes, does not a nutritionist-physician make.

THE FOLLY OF FOOD GROUPS

I sometimes wonder where did the notion of including dairy and meats in the four *basic* food groups come from? Meat is not a part of the food in the Hindu culture, clearly one of the oldest and most durable among the cultures of the world. Dairy is excluded from the foods of many people in the Far East, a circumstance that reflects a considered position based on their understanding of the relationship between food and the human condition rather than a ritualistic abstinence. How did dairy and meat earn the right to be included among the four basic groups in America? The answer is that here in America foods become *great* only when the smart money says they are great. And the dairy and meat industries in the United States. have a lot of smart money.

Cow's milk is an excellent food for a baby cow. Man is the only living organism that drinks milk all his life, and not of his own mother. In my choice of beverages which follows in this chapter, I include cow's milk in Choice Three drinks and goat's milk among Choice Two Beverages. Why do I include cow's milk in Choice Three beverages? Because cow's milk is a highly allergenic food. We are taught that milk is essential for our children. We are told by the "experts" on the payroll of the dairy industry that milk is *the* best source of calcium. Nothing could be further from truth. I have cared for a very large number of children who were literally raised on antibiotics for throat and ear infections. Almost all of these children were allergic, and most of them were allergic to milk. Diagnosis and treatment of their food allergy and incompatibilities and mold allergy followed by nutrient therapy restored the integrity of their molecular defenses. We were able to completely avoid the use of antibiotics in most of these children. If the cow's milk is an excellent food for baby cows, then goat's milk must be an excellent food for baby goats? Why is goat's milk included among Choice Two beverages? The difference between the cow's milk and the goat's milk is frequency of drinking. Allergic individuals become allergic to cow's milk because they drink it every day. Indeed if a person with food allergy drinks goat's milk every day, he will very likely become allergic to goat's milk.

If we cannot go by the conventional wisdom about a balanced diet and the RDA experts, what are we to do? The answer is really quite simple: We must turn to the labor of learning, understanding and *knowing*. My discussion of the basic chemistry of life, life span and aging-oxidant molecules in the early part of this chapter is a good beginning.

Supermarket foods cause obesity. This stands to common sense. These foods are usually rich in oxidized and denatured fats, loaded with salt, and laced with toxic byproducts of food processing. All three factors lead to buildup of excess fats in fat cells. It is well-known that Europeans consume larger quantities of butter and cold-pressed oils, which contain unoxidized and un-denatured fats, than we Americans. From this one would expect that obesity should be a much smaller problem for Europeans than it is for us Americans. This indeed is true. It is a common observation for those who frequently travel in both continents. Of course, Europe is being rapidly polluted with industrial and agricultural toxicants. Also, it is being invaded by the American fast food industry with French fries laced with salt and soaked with toxic fats. And with its milk shakes and cheeseburgers. Given time, severe obesity will be as common in Europe as it is in America, unless we all wake up to these destructive trends.

I am not aware if the above observation about obesity patterns in the United States and Europe has been documented with any statistical studies. What is well-established with statistical studies is similar phenomena in experimental animals. Studies have shown that when two groups of rats are offered cafeteria-type and natural foods with equivalent caloric value, rats eating cafeteria-type foods become obese while those in the natural group do not (*Clin Endocrinol Metab* 13:437;1984).

Similarly rats offered sugar-rich fluids get "addicted" to sugar (much like our children do) and become obese (*Fed Proc* 36:154; 1977). Needless to say, rats offered fat-rich diets become obese (*J Nutr* 102:1187; 1972).

Life span nutrition is a study of our foods and their relationship to our lives. Life span nutrition is about knowing food and the way it sustains life or truncates it. The key word in this statement is *knowing*. There are three steps in life span nutrition. First, we learn about foods. Next, we understand the difference between foods that sustain us and the materials with which we stuff our bowels but which do not preserve our health. Third, and this can come to us only after we learn and understand our foods, is *knowing* the relationship between our food and our lives.

LIFE SPAN AND AGING-OXIDANT FOODS

In our simplified life chemistry language, we may use the term life span foods for foods that support the life span molecules. These, as I indicated earlier, are molecules that nature designed to assure that all living things can live their normal life spans in good health. Aging-oxidant foods, by contrast, are foods which support the aging-oxidant molecules, the molecules that nature designed to age all living things and make sure no form of life lives forever. The balance between the life span and aging-oxidant molecules is the essential chemical equation of life.

In this monograph I include lists of beverages and foods that I have divided into four categories: three categories of life span foods and one category of aging-oxidizing choices. These categories are intended to show the relative nutritional values and desirability of these food items from a life span perspective. I give below the specific *molecular, electromagnetic, empirical, and clinical* criteria I use to divide foods and beverages into these four groups. I have carefully examined the ancient as well as well as current literature describing the empirical observations about the healthful and adverse effects of foods and beverages on human health and disease. I have had extensive personal experience with micro-elisa blood test and electrodermal conductance technology for detection of food incompatibility and allergy and abnormal bowel responses to food. I discuss this subject further in the chapter On Limbic Eating. Above all, I have been guided by the principal of holistic molecular relatedness in human biology. The knowledge of the structure and function of individual nutrient molecules must be integrated with the known molecular dynamics of health and disease in an holistic fashion, and from a long-term life span perspective.

Five Essentials of Life-Span Foods

First,

the life span foods must support the full life span of the individual. These foods should do so in one or more of the following four ways: 1) provide food substances that are composed of life span molecules; 2) provide food substances that support life span molecules; 3) provide substances that neutralize aging-oxidant molecules that threaten life span molecules; and 4) provide substances that serve as fuel and building materials for various body tissues without causing undue oxidative stress.

Second,

the life span foods must be able to prevent or suppress a host of molecular roller coasters that generate AOMs or destroy LSMs and so cause disease. These include rapid bursts of oxidative molecules (oxyradicals and other free radicals), rapid acidotic shifts, sharp hypoglycemic-hyperglycemic shifts, quick releases of catecholamine surges (adrenaline and its cousin molecules), large cholinergic pulses, and sudden fluctuations in neurotransmitter levels.

Third,

the life span foods must fully support the internal ecology of the bowel. These foods must facilitate the digestive and absorptive processes in the bowel, and sustain the normal bowel flora. Further, the life span foods should restore the bowel transit time, bowel perfusion (blood supply), Ph (acid-alkaline) changes and digestive enzymatic functions.

Fourth,

the life span foods must not trigger allergic food reactions and abnormal bowel responses to foods. Evidently, foods that cause allergic and incompatibility reactions and abnormal bowel responses for a person are powerful aging-oxidant foods for *him even though they may be life span foods for others.* Food incompatibility is a paradox: It is a complex subjects full of inconsistencies for physicians who do not receive the necessary training for diagnosis and management of food allergy; and it is a patently simple matter for physicians who make the necessary effort to become familiar with the diversity of clinical symptoms and patterns of suffering caused by it. To properly diagnose and manage food allergy, we need knowledgeable professionals and accurate testing procedures. See the Appendix for a listing of professional organizations devoted to environmental and nutritional medicine.

Fifth,

the life span foods must bring the total caloric intake to a level consistent with the level of physical activity. Strong clinical and experimental evidence supports the viewpoint that caloric restriction is necessary for living a full life span. People often think of achieving this by limiting the caloric intake. I prefer to achieve the optimal balance between caloric intake and physical activity by focusing on limbic exercise rather than by dieting.

Supporting the Life Span Molecules

We will compare freshly squeezed vegetable juice with a commercial preparation of a mixed vegetable juice. I urge the reader to do the following simple experiment to test the validity of this example. Open a can of vegetable juice and prepare a glass of freshly squeezed vegetable juice with red beets, carrots and celery. Take a sip of the fresh juice. Wait for a few moments. Next take a sip of the commercial canned juice. Repeat the two steps a few times at intervals of one to two minutes. Now let us compare the two. The fresh juice has a "life sense" to it. It is fresh, true, tasteful, invigorating and life-giving. The canned juice is flat, tasteless and carries a sense of staleness. Most people will *know* the truth of these statements the very first time they put them to the test.

Taste is an acquired sense. This means that this simple experiment clearly carries a bias *in favor of the canned vegetable juice* because most people drink canned vegetable juice and have an acquired taste for such juice. Fresh juice made up of uncommonly eaten vegetables for most people can be expected to be a "new" and hence an unfamiliar taste. Yet, despite this bias, fresh juice will unequivocally emerge as the clear winner. Why? It is a matter of the *wisdom* of our taste buds and our digestive-absorptive cells.

Our taste buds know more than our calculating and computing minds. Our digestive-absorptive cells know more than our most profound insights into the workings of nature. In the language of chemistry, life *is* living enzymes. The fresh juices are living juices. These juices live because their enzymes live.

The canned juices are dead juices. These juices are dead because their enzymes are dead. Our taste buds know this even after years of having been molested by dead and dying foods.

The fresh vegetable juice wins the contest because our taste buds have not forgotten the difference between the life-sustaining life span enzymes that give fresh foods the life sense and the aging-oxidant molecules that accumulate in processed foods, rendering them flat and lifeless. Our taste buds retain a clear memory of what is life-giving and what is lifeless. See the section on vegetable fasting in the chapter On Limbic Eating.

Life span of foods and profitability of our food industry are sworn enemies of each other.

What determines the life span of foods? The food enzymes. What assures the profitability of our food industry? Long shelf lives of foods. How are the shelf lives of food prolonged? By food processing and by using food preservatives. How do food processing and food preservatives work? By destroying the food enzymes.

What is contained in our commercial canned foods? Money-making dreams of our marketing moguls. What is carried in our "preserved" foods, life span foods or aging-oxidant foods? The profitability in food products, the money men of food industry know, is in the shelf life of food items. What they do not seem to recognize — or do not care to know — is that the shelf-life of foods is inversely proportional to their life span. The money men of our food industry lace their vegetable juices with salt, up to 600 to 800 mg per can, to assure that their juices do not spoil. The salt kills the life enzymes of their juices. A dead juice cannot get any deader. A juice is now preserved. What is really preserved is the profitability of juice canners.

FOODS THAT FUEL MOLECULAR ROLLER COASTERS

What happens to the sugar metabolism of a child when he gulps a can of soda or a glass of orange juice in three minutes? This question arose in my mind some years ago during a lecture to the medical staff of Holy Name Hospital. I was presenting data for a series of over 1000 glucose tolerance tests performed in our laboratory that I personally studied. Among patients who developed symptoms during the glucose tolerance study, 9 out of every 10 developed symptoms when their blood glucose levels rose rapidly within the first half hour. The remaining 10% individuals developed symptoms when the blood levels became low near the end of the study period. The slide projected on the slide made two telling point for me. First, that the symptoms evidently were caused by sudden increases in the blood levels rather than by low blood sugar levels as is generally believed. Second, the symptoms experienced by these individuals were identical to those caused by excess adrenaline and related stress hormones.

Let us consider what happens to a child when he rapidly drinks a glass of orange juice or a can or soda. The blood glucose in health ranges from 75 to 105 mg/ 100 ml. We will take the example of an eight-year-old girl with a blood sugar level of 100 mg/100 ml (or 1,000 mg/1,000 ml or 1 gram per liter of blood). The total volume of circulating blood in our girl will be approximately 4 liters. This means the total amount of glucose circulating in her blood is 4 grams. Since one level teaspoon of sugar holds 4 grams of sugar, she has just one teaspoonful of sugar circulating in the blood in her *entire* body. A can of soda contains from 7 to 9 teaspoons of sugar. For this example, we say that our girl drinks her can of soda in 10 minutes. Now let us add it up. In a period of 10 minutes, she pours 7 to 9 times as much sugar into her blood as exists in the circulating blood in her *total* body. What does this avalanche of sugar do to her sugar metabolism?

Rapid shifts in the blood sugar levels are accompanied by equally rapid surges in the secretion of insulin and adrenaline and its cousin molecules. These, in turn, are associated with sudden, highly stressful changes in the blood and tissue levels of neurotransmitter and other messenger molecules. The result: the whole biology is thrown into turmoil.

SUPPORT FOR THE NORMAL BOWEL ECOLOGY

For many years I have studied a host of clinical syndromes in which the symptom-complexes can be related to events occurring in the bowel. As a hospital pathologist, I have examined more than 11,000 bowel biopsies during the last 25 years. During the early 1980s, my research colleague, Madhava Ramanarayanan, Ph.D., and I first introduced the use of micro-elisa technology for allergy diagnosis and analyzed thousands of blood specimens for food and inhalant allergy. As a practitioner of molecular medicine, I have had the opportunity to care for a very large number of patients with chronic bowel disorders. This work has given me some valuable insights into the nature of chronic bowel disorders and the special restorative capacity of some life span foods. I include below some text from my monograph *The Altered Bowel Ecology States and Health Preservation* published by the Institute of Preventive Medicine, Denville, New Jersey.

The human molecular defenses exist as plants rooted in the soil of the bowel contents.

The ancients seemed to have known this intuitively. We seem to have taken a very circuitous route to this most fundamental of all aspects of the immune system.

A cell looks at the world around it through its cell membrane. It is the cell membrane that separates internal order from external order for the cell. In my monograph, *The Agony and the Death of a Cell* published in the 1991 syllabus of the American Academy of Environmental Medicine, I discuss at length the energy and biochemical events that occur at the cell membrane in health and disease. I also discuss the evolution of molecular host defense mechanisms, both of immune and non-immune types, in various life-forms as they differentiate from simple single-cell forms to multicellular forms to highly developed complex organisms. But the fundamental pattern of host defenses has remained the same: The cell membrane or its counterparts carry the primary responsibility of preserving the biologic integrity of the organisms. For man, gut mucosa is the true counterpart of the cell membrane of the unicellular organisms. From a phylogenetic perspective, the gut mucosa would be expected to be the primary host defense organ. This indeed is the case when one looks at the health and disease issues for man from a *holistic* perspective.

The following foods stand out in their restorative value for people with disrupted internal ecology of the bowel: burdock, daikon, garlic, ginger, radish, sea vegetables, pre-digested soy products, squashes, turnips and some herbal products that can be taken as food supplements. Some other foods favor the overgrowth of yeast and some other pathogenic bacteria in the bowel, and so are best avoided in the altered states of bowel ecology. These foods include foods that are rich in simple sugars, contain yeast products, or have a high content of fermented items.

Food Compatibility and Allergy

The subjects of food incompatibility and allergy and abnormal bowel responses to foods are essential subjects. In the prevailing notions of drug medicine in America, these subjects are considered materials for the fringe physicians. Scientists in medicine, I often hear, must stay clear of such hucksterism. I sometime wonder if there is another area in medicine in which more irresponsible statements are made by otherwise responsible physicians than in this area. A great enigma for me is this: How can any physician engage in any healing art without making nutrition the centerpiece of his practice? After all, as I wrote earlier, we are made of food, are sustained by food, fall ill when we eat wrong foods, and die if food is withheld from us.

What is food for one is poison for another, observed Hippocrates almost 2,500 years ago. Hippocrates, it seems, learned his lesson from the Man from the Rift Valley who observed that some foods were healing and some others made him sick. We physicians are the intellectual progeny of this Man from Africa, even though many of us are now infatuated with drugs and despise the word empiricism.

What is the commonest cause of fatigue after eating? Milk allergy. Is egg an excellent food? Yes. Should every one eat eggs? No. Egg is a very allergenic food. People with allergic genes are very likely to be allergic to eggs. Which is a better food for some one with allergic nasal and sinus symptoms, wheat or wild rice? Wild rice, because allergy to wild rice is very uncommon while wheat is one of the major allergens.

The subjects of food allergy and abnormal bowel responses to foods are of paramount importance for both people who suffer from chronic immune disorders and professionals who care for them. It is also a complex subject. Food allergy often causes chronic headaches, arthritis, colitis, asthma, disorders of mood, memory and mentation, and hyperactivity in children. In the prevailing mode of drug medicine, these afflictions are usually treated with drugs. Food allergy as the true cause remains undiagnosed. The proper diagnosis and management of food allergy requires electrodermal conductance tests and micro-elisa blood tests (or skin tests). In my view, the electrodermal methods in the hands of experienced professionals give a far superior total profile of food tolerance and intolerance than the blood tests. As the benefits of this technology become better known to the physician community, it will, despite some variability in test results caused by individual operators, become widely accepted for this purpose.

EATING LESS TO SUPPORT THE FULL LIFE SPAN

It is now clearly established in experimental animals that ad lib eating shortens the species life span. I discuss this subject at length in the chapter, On Limbic eating. What causes sugar craving? What are the causes of overeating? Sugar causes sugar craving. Rarely do we realize that more than sugar, salt causes sugar craving. What brings on gorging-starving-gorging cycles? The catabolic maladaptation.I discuss these questions at length in the chapters On the Nature of Obesity, The Catabolic Maladaptation and Why Dieting Cannot work. Here I make one important point: It is extremely difficult, if not impossible, to eat less for vitality and for living the full life span in optimal health if we eat aging-oxidant foods. Aging-oxidant foods create molecular roller coasters that cause food craving and lead to paralyzing eating- bingeing cycles. Aging-oxidant foods cause catabolic maladaptation which trap the overweight person much like the skylight over our patio trapped the butterfly.

FOUR CRITICAL ASPECTS OF LIFE SPAN NUTRITION

First, we are what we observe.

The ancients believed that we are what we eat. They knew, intuitively it seems, that we are our food and our food is us. They seem to have known what their food was and how it affected them. Our problems today are different. We neither know what our food is nor understand how it affects us. Does a man eating a lunch of cheeseburger, French fries and milk shake know what is in his food? Does he know how such food will affect him? Does he ever try to *observe* the relationship between his food and himself? Optimal nutrition for the life span of an individual requires that he learn to observe how his food responds to him and how he responds to his food.

Second, bowel is the most important defense organ of the body.

Human molecular defenses exist as plants rooted in the soil of the bowel contents. The bowel is the primary interface between the world within us and that outside our skin. Altered bowel ecology states are the dominant chronic disorder of our time. Recent research clearly shows what the ancients seemed to recognize intuitively: that the human bowel is the primary seat of our molecular defenses against disease. Molecular events in the bowel determine whether we stay healthy or get sick. Immune cells (T cells, B cells and Killer lymphocyte cells) are of secondary importance in the integrity of the immune system. Changes in the number and function of these immune cells occur late in the continuum of health, dis-ease and disease. Antibodies, lymphokines and related molecules produced by these cells are messenger molecules. The events that initiate and perpetuate immune dysfunctions are *molecular events that occur in the bowel.* Life span nutrition requires that we understand what our bowel ecology is and how it is preserved.

Third, injured foods injure tissues.

Food items, like people and plants, have defined life spans. The life span of food items, like that of people and plants, is determined by the equilibrium between the food LSMs and food AOMs. This equilibrium sets the rate of oxidation of that particular food. In other words, foods, like people, have their own redox potential. Aging (spoiling) of foods is caused by their own oxidative mechanisms. Foods have built-in mechanisms for controlling their oxidative pathways. To illustrate, lettuce is rich in vitamin C, but it can lose up to 80 % of its vitamin C if it is finely chopped and exposed to oxygen in air.

Our foods are badly injured. We injure our plant foods when we injure our food chains. We injure our plants with fertilizers, herbicides and pesticides. We injure our animal foods with antibiotics and steroids. We injure our foods with processing. We injure our foods with preservatives. What is not good for bugs cannot be much good for us.

Fourth, we must respect our food if our food is to respect us.

To be able to respect our food, we must first *know* it. To know it, we must first learn and understand it. To learn and understand it, we need two things: the science of food and the common sense test. "Food science" alone is not enough. I cite some examples in the chapter, On Limbic Eating. Bad numbers are driving good sense out of our nutrition, just as they do to our medicine. This is true of many of the so-called research studies published in some of the most prestigious medical journals in this country. The acid test of common sense must be accepted as the true test of what is right and what is not in nutrition.

Nutrition Researchers, Nutrition "Experts," Nutrition Enthusiasts and Nutrition Philosophers

Nutrition researchers are people who study the effect of one nutrient at any time and carefully define the molecular structure and function of individual nutrients. Nutrition experts, I mention earlier, are people who put mice or medical students on some diet for a few weeks, produce and publish their numbers, never try to reverse health disorders with nutritional protocols and call all those who try to do so quacks. Nutrition enthusiasts are those who are fascinated with one nutrient and ascribe all types of health benefits to it. Their belief is usually based on some bit of sound molecular knowledge. These enthusiasts consume large quantities of their favorite foods in the hope of supplying themselves with their favorite nutrients, usually with limited benefits. Nutrition philosophers think holistically. They have a much wider perspective. They see, and are guided by, the holistic molecular relatedness in human biology.

The work of our nutrition researchers about the structure and function of nutrient molecules must be treasured. They give us the *true* science of nutrition. Our nutrition philosophers must be honored and heeded. They give us the larger vision of health and the human condition. Our nutrition enthusiasts should be tolerated, for they may be the future nutrition philosophers. Perhaps some of them may even become future nutrition scientists. We have no use for our nutrition experts, who practice drug medicine, consider nutrients of no value in treatment of disease , and look down upon those who practice nutritional as quacks.

ANTIOXIDANT ENTHUSIASTS

Antioxidant enthusiasts have good "molecular" reasons for their enthusiasm. They point to studies that show that mosquitoes and other insects live longer if they are fed antioxidants. Aging is widely believed to be the result of molecular injury caused by free radicals that in turn are produced by oxidative molecular injury. Another theory of aging considers protein cross-linking as the basic chemical reaction of the aging process. The proponents of this theory point out that cross-linking of proteins is primarily caused by free radicals. This also supports the viewpoint of antioxidant enthusiasts. *The fundamental nature of the aging process, I indicated earlier, is the spontaneity of the process of oxidation in nature.* Oxidation in nature is a spontaneous process. It does not require expenditure of energy.

Antioxidant enthusiasts have sound scientific reasons for their enthusiasm. We must, however, recognize that there is little conceptual difference between drug therapy for symptom suppression and antioxidant therapy to reverse oxidant damage. Both approaches build dams downstream and attempt to make the water flow upstream. We need life span strategies to prevent the need for accelerated molecular oxidative damage. This requires effective self-regulatory methods that down-regulate the metabolic oxidative stress.

NIACIN ENTHUSIASTS

Niacin enthusiast believe that niacin is a great "energy" and "cholesterol-lowering" vitamin. Indeed, niacin plays important roles in molecular events that generate energy, and may be rightfully regarded as an electron transfer vitamin. Niacin also lowers blood cholesterol levels. So we cannot simply dismiss their claims. However, we need to remember that prolonged, unsupervised niacin therapy has been known to cause liver injury.

OXYGEN ENTHUSIASTS

Oxygen is essential for life. The oxygen enthusiasts consider this to be the final truth in human biology. There are many types of bio-oxidative therapies in vogue. Many of them do give good short-term results. How can we disagree with the oxygen enthusiasts? Or can we? Oxygen is a molecular Dr.

Jekyll and Mr. Hyde. The oxygen enthusiasts understand the Dr. Jekyll role of oxygen but do not seem to know the Mr. Hyde side of the oxygen story. Oxygen ushers life in. Oxygen sustains life. The oxygen enthusiasts know this. Oxygen also terminates life. Oxidant enthusiasts do not know this.

PANTETHEINE AND CYSTEINE ENTHUSIASTS

These nutrients are powerful life span molecules. Pantetheine is necessary for production of another molecule called Co-enzyme A which is essential for energy generation. Pantetheine enthusiasts consider themselves "energy people," hence their infatuation with pantetheine. Cysteine is a part of methionine-cysteine-taurine complex, which plays a critical antioxidant role in human life processes. It is easy to see why cysteine enthusiasts worship their deity.

OMEGA-3 AND OMEGA-6 ENTHUSIASTS

Omega-3 and omega-6 oils are required for production of essential fatty acids. Essential fatty acids, of course, are called *essential* because they are essential for the health of all cells in the body. These fatty acids are essential for the structural and functional integrity of plasma membranes of cells and for production of almost all hormones. Furthermore, these acids are source molecules for all the prostaglandins and leukotrienes that are essential for our molecular defenses. I discuss this subject at length in my monograph *Choua, Cholesterol Cats and Chelation.*

MAGNESIUM ENTHUSIASTS

I must confess I am very reverential to magnesium.

Life began on our planet Earth with conversion of solar energy into chemical bond energy. Chemical bond energy is the thread which holds together the posies of life form flowers. Chlorophyll converts solar energy into chemical bond energy and is a magnesium chelate.

ATPase and Acetyl CoA are premium molecules in human energy dynamics. Magnesium is a cofactor for both.

Methionine-homocysteine-cysteine-taurine and cysteine-glutathione sulfhydryl systems are essential life preserving anti-oxidant defenses of the body. These pathways are magnesium dependent.

The first step in glucose metabolism is conversion of glucose to glucose-6-phosphate. This reaction requires hexokinase which is a magnesium-dependent enzyme.

Delta-6-desaturase is a critical enzyme in the conversion of fatty acids of plant and animal origin into longer chains and unsaturated fatty acids essential for human metabolism. Delta-6-desaturase is a magnesium dependent enzyme.

Magnesium serves as a cofactor in diverse reactions involved in DNA and protein synthesis.

Magnesium is essential for many enzymatic reactions that use vitamin B_1 (thiamine) and vitamin B_6 (pyridoxine). These vitamins, in turn, are required for biosynthesis of essential neurotransmitter such as serotonin, GABA (gamma-amino-butyric acid) and melatonin.

Magnesium is a cofactor for the metabolism of yet other neurotransmitter such as acetylcholine.

Increased intracellular levels of calcium poison cellular enzymes, hence the fascination of our drug industry with calcium channel blockers. Magnesium is nature's calcium channel blocker.

Magnesium serves as a cofactor in many biochemical reactions that are involved the maintenance of intracellular concentration of other cations such as potassium, sodium and calcium. Magnesium is also a cofactor for a large number of enzymes such as kinases.

Acutely ill hospitalized patients almost always become magnesium-poor within a few days. Such deficiency almost always goes unrecognized because we continue to insist that a deficiency state must be documented with blood tests before embarking upon magnesium replacement therapy. The fact that only less than 1% of total body magnesium exists in the blood does not seem important to us (skeletal and intracellular compartments contain approximately 53% and 46% of magnesium respectively). We fail to see the obvious: Increased oxidant stress on cell membranes associated with illness and resulting in hospitalization leads to leakage of magnesium out of the cell and into the extracellular space. In addition, it masks the intracellular magnesium deficiency.

The ideal test for functional magnesium deficiency, in my judgment, is an intravenous therapeutic trial.

It is my clinical observation that oral magnesium supplements frequently fail to replenish magnesium stores within the cells. In patients with chronic fatigue, myalgia, fibromyositis, and persistent muscle spasms and pain, oral magnesium supplements often give poor results while intravenous magnesium therapy almost always gives rapid and satisfactory clinical benefits. The same holds for patients with asthma, irregular heart rhythm, and severe backache. I once used intravenous magnesium along with other micronutrients for one of my patients with severe depression in a desperate — and fortunately successful — attempt to avoid hospitalization (this patient had very traumatic memory of previous hospital admission for depression). Indeed, there is extensive evidence that disorders of mood, memory and mentation, and psychiatric symptoms such as confusion, disorientation, agitation and depression are common in magnesium-deficient patient (*JAMA* 224:1749; 1973).

Magnesium is often poorly absorbed; clinical studies indicate absorption rate ranging from 50% to 70% in healthy subjects on normal diet (Shils, M.E. in *Modern nutrition in health and disease* Philadelphia: Lea & Fibiger, pp. 159-192). The intestinal absorption of magnesium is further decreased in magnesium-deficient states (*Intern. J. Neuroscience* 61:87; 1991). Indeed, correction of magnesium deficiency in many patients is so problematic that a genetic basis for reduced magnesium absorption has been considered (*Cecil Textbook of Medicine 1988*).

I know my advice to use intravenous magnesium drip as a test for functional magnesium deficiency in states of accelerated oxidative stress will rankle many of my colleagues in mainstream medicine. *I stand by my recommendation.* It is one of the *most* valuable diagnostic tool for the clinician caring for people with unremitting suffering. I refer the professional reader to my review article *Magnesium and Oxidative Cell Membrane Injury* that appeared in the spring 1992 issue of *The Environmental Physician* published by the American Academy of Environmental Medicine, Denver, Colorado.

HOLISTIC MOLECULAR RELATEDNESS
IN HUMAN BIOLOGY

Human biology is an ever changing kaleidoscope of molecular mosaics. No nutrients can exist or do its work all by itself. Nutrient depend upon each other. This is the essence of what I call the principle of holistic molecular relatedness in human biology. Let us consider some examples.

Taurine, an amino acid, is a great "magnesium saver" molecule. Magnesium, a mineral, is necessary for delta-6-desaturase. Delta-6, an enzyme, is essential for conversation of fatty acids linoleic and linolenic acids into arachidonic acid (AA). AA, a fatty acid, is a precursor of prostaglandins. Prostaglandins, essential hormones, communicate with cell receptors. Cell receptors, the "molecular gofers", activate mRNA. mRNA, a messenger molecule, carries the "sales order" to DNA polymerase. DNA polymerase use the DNA molecules as templates to make genes. Genes regulated protein synthesis. Protein synthesis requires amino acids. Human metabolism goes looking for taurine. The cycle goes on. One small molecular mosaic is completed.

A common practice is to find out which food contains large quantities of a given nutrient of interest and then consume large quantities of that food. This simplistic notion conflicts with the fundamental principle of holistic molecular relatedness in human biology. This practice is not advisable if our goal is optimal health for the full life span.

Life Span Food and Beverage Choices

Choice One Foods and Beverages

Food choices in this category are the best. These foods are ideal for sustaining a life span in optimal health, and meet my four criteria for life span foods (when allergy to any of these foods for an individual has been excluded). These items are excellent sources of steady-state energy and essential nutrients. Choice One foods are least likely to cause allergic reactions, least likely to trigger molecular roller coasters, least likely to increase acidotic stresses, and are least likely to cause absorptive and digestive dysfunctions.

Choice One Foods may be eaten in rotation as frequently as three to four times a week. I reiterate for emphasis that no food should be eaten every day of the week.

Choice Two Foods and Beverages

Food choices in this second category are second-best food choices. These food items are good sources of steady-state energy and nutrients (when food allergy has been excluded). Needless to say, these items fall somewhere between the Choice One and Choice Three foods. These foods may also be eaten frequently and in rotation, two to three times a week, but not every day.

Choice Three Foods and Beverages

Food choices in this category should be rotated on the basis of once every three or four days. This recommendation is based upon a careful assessment of the impact of these foods on the several life span issues discussed above. For instance, egg is included in Choice Three Foods. Eggs are an excellent source of first-class proteins and phospholipid which are so essential for cellular health. The primary reason for including eggs in Choice Three category is food allergy. Eggs rank high among the list of foods that cause serious allergy. Macrobiotics folks completely restrict eggs which, in my judgment, unnecessarily excludes an excellent food from the diet of people who are not allergic to it. Some low-carbohydrate, high-fat diet enthusiasts promote daily consumption of eggs. This, in my judgment, unnecessarily increases the risk of food allergy. We become allergic to foods we eat most commonly. I might add here that the incidence of food allergy is rising at an alarming rate because of progressive oxidant stress on our biology caused by environmental pollutants.

It is important to rotate foods in Choice Three category. I recommend a three- or four-day rotation even when food allergy does not exist.

Food allergy is of two types: fixed food allergy and cyclical food allergy. In fixed food allergy, the individual develops unmistakable allergic reactions, often serious and within several minutes, each time he eats that food. Example: hives after eating shrimp. Fixed food allergy is much less common than cyclical food allergy. In cyclical food allergy, the reactions may occur anytime during a five-day period after the food is ingested. Furthermore, the reactions are often unclear to the uninitiated. Example: fatigue, mood swings and inability to concentrate after eating the food.

In my own experience, a vast majority of those with cyclical food allergy can eat the allergic foods after proper treatment and when the foods are eaten in a four-day rotation. This point is of considerable practical importance. People with food allergy are often allergic to common foods such as dairy, wheat, egg, corn, beef, orange, lettuce, baker's yeast and brewer's yeast. It is very difficult to avoid all these foods for long.

Life Span and Aging-Oxidant Beverages

An optimal state of hydration is essential for optimal health.

Most of us, when not making a conscious effort, stay in a state of mild dehydration. Dehydration stresses our metabolic pathways, and in particular exaggerates the acidotic stress caused by our food and our environments. In general, aging-oxidant foods increase the dehydration stress and life span foods diminish it. A simple remedy for the metabolic problems of dehydration and acidosis is a habit of drinking life span fluids.

A drink of eight ounces of one of the life span fluids is desirable every three to four hours except during the late evening and night hours.

First, we need to learn about life span and aging-oxidant fluids. In the life span terminology used in this book, all fluids which increase the rates of oxidative molecular injury are regarded as aging-oxidant fluids. Examples are fluids that contain stimulants such as caffeine and nicotine, environmental pollutants and other agents that disrupt normal steady-state metabolism such as alcohol. Following are some suggestions about taking in life span fluids and avoiding or minimizing aging-oxidant fluids.

Life Span Choices

Spring and mineral waters
Vegetable juices, fresh, unsalted
    (carrot, daikon, spinach, beets, celery)
Bancha, barley and Mu teas
Grain coffee
Yannoh (a coffee substitute made from barley, rye and chicory)
Gingerroot water (cheapest and best water. Boil one and half
        inch of fresh gingerroot with one gallon of water, let it
        cool, transfer it into a glass bottle discarding the last one
        inch of water behind, and refrigerate. Ginger alkaloids
        bind to water pollutants and precipitate them down).

Herbal teas, in rotation and as prescribed by a professional.
Herbal teas should be rotated as beverages as well as for

their healthful effects. These teas are not recommended as treatment of specific active diseases except under the direct supervision of a physician.

Fruit teas: almond, cherries, and others

Second Line Choices

Fruit juices (A large glass of orange juice may contain as many as 6-8 teaspoons of fructose which is metabolized somewhat slower than glucose, still it causes a sugar overload.

Lime, lemon and light colas are caffeine-free and have citrate (alkaline effect) and should be preferred to dark sodas (which contain caffeine and phosphate).

Aspartame: acceptable on occasions except for people with aspartame sensitivity (molecular individuality)

Aging-Oxidant Beverages

Black (common) tea

Coffee

Dark colas are caffeine-rich, contain phosphates and are better avoided (or restricted).

Alcoholic beverages

(Alcohol is an aging-oxidant molecule. However, when taken in modest amounts on special family and other occasions, it has some redeeming desirable effects on mood.)

Life Span and Aging-Oxidant Teas

Life span (LS) teas are herbal beverages that support life span molecules. Aging-oxidant (AO) teas are beverages that favor aging-oxidant molecules.

Tea appears to have been first used in Assam. Buddhists carried it to the Far East, the British to the West. The tea plant is a nourishing plant. How we make use of this plant determines whether we obtain a LS beverage or an AO beverage.

Black tea (common tea) is an AO tea. It is acidic, caffeine-rich and favors the aging-oxidant molecules. It decreases tissue levels of some life span enzymes such as transketolase, lactic dehydrogenase and thiamin diphosphatase (Experientia 45:112; 1989). Green tea is milder than black tea, is acidic, favors AOMs, and hence is an AO tea. Bancha tea (late-growing tea) is alkaline and caffeine-free. It protects the stomach lining from acidotic stress, preserves normal gastric ecology, promotes digestion, and hence is an LS tea. Common coffee (from coffee beans) is acidic and caffeine-rich (up to 80 mg of caffeine per cup). Decaffeinated coffee has much lower levels of caffeine (3-10 mg per cup) but is acidic and often contains residual methylene chloride and ethyl acetate, chemicals that many tea companies use to decaffeinate their tea.

Grain teas (barley, brown rice, millet, corn-silk) are neutral-to-alkaline, caffeine-free life span teas. These teas restore gastric and bowel ecology, and have several known mild medicinal effects. Mu tea is a popular blend that contains ginseng and several other herbs. It is an alkaline, caffeine-free life span tea.

Herbal Teas

Specific individual herbal teas listed below have several established biochemical medicinal effects and their regular use for specific health disorders should be physician-supervised.

Chamomile flower: Egyptians used it to slow the aging process.
Golden seal root: general life span tea. Biblical Rx, American Indian Rx
Echinacea root: general life span tea.
Astragalus: general life span
Linden flower: general life span tea
Ginseng root: general life span tea
Peau D'Arco inner bark: for altered bowel ecology states*
Flax seeds tea: for lung and bowel ecology
Comfrey roots and leaves: for stomach and bowel ecology
Caraway seeds: for stomach and bowel ecology
Thyme leaves: for stomach and bowel ecology (pronounced "time")
Cascara sagrada: for bowel ecology
Peppermint: for stomach ecology
Alfalfa leaves and seeds: for stomach ecology
Clover blossoms: for liver disorders
Juniper berry: for bladder ecology
Horsetail: for hair, skin and nail ecology
Valerian root: for nervous system disorders (Latin *valere*=well-being)
Huckleberry: for hypoglycemia and hyperglycemia
Hawthorn flower and berries: for hypertension and heart disease
Rose petal tea for eyestrain.
Black oats (with whiskers) tea for anxiety.
Marigold petal tea for anxiety.
Sage tea for flu-like symptoms.
Gingerroot: gastric and bowel ecology; for motion sickness
Feverfew leaves: for chronic headache (also freeze dried in tablets)
Aloe vera gel: for bowel ecology. Taken as syrup or gel.
* See my monograph *The Altered States of Bowel Ecology and Health Preservation* for a discussion of how normal bowel ecology is damaged by antibiotics, drugs, toxic foods and stress and how it can be restored with

nutrient and herbal therapies.

Beverages

First Choice	Second Choice	Third Choice
LS waters*	Spring waters	Skim milk, cow**
Vegetable juices***	Deep well water	Low-fat milk, cow
Ginger water	Mineral waters	Dark sodas
Bancha tea	Fruit teas	Orange juice
Mu tea	Grapefruit juice	Sweet fruit juices
Barley tea	Apple juice	Cranberry juice
Grain coffee	Soy milk, diluted	Salted vegetable juices
Herbal teas****	Rice milk, diluted	Nut milks, diluted
	Light sodas, diet	Coconut juice
	Goat milk	
	Buffalo milk	

* The ideal drinking water is a fresh, natural, nonchlorinated spring or deep well water obtained from natural, noncommercial sources. (Problem: where are we to find such water?) Bottled spring waters generally go through a packaging process: Some are good; others are not.

** Cow's milk appears in the third category for reason of its allergenicity.

*** The best vegetable juices are fresh unsalted juices. Cans of most commercially available vegetable juices contain as much as 500-600 mg of sodium (a "life span mineral" turned into an "aging-oxidant mineral" by the American food industry). Unsalted canned vegetable juices are next best choices. See the section on fasting in the chapter On Limbic Eating.

**** Herbal teas are excellent choices but must be taken in rotation and under the supervision of a knowledgeable professional. One or two teaspoons of food grade glycerine may be added to herbal teas as a sweetener.

Aging-Oxidant Beverages

Coffee	Tea (common black)	Coca
Chocolate	Malt drinks	Ice cream sodas
Milk shakes	Alcohol *	

* Alcohol in small amounts has some good physiological effects and other positive effects on mood and spirits. These effects, as I wrote earlier, may indeed counterbalance the essential aging-oxidant effects of alcohol. Thus, complete abstinence, except in the case of persons with past or present dependence on it, is not essential.

Fats and Oils

First Choice	Second Choice	Third choice
Olive oil	Safflower oil	Corn oil
Ghee *	Sunflower oil	Palm oil
Butter	Soybean oil	Peanut oil
Sesame oil	Avocado oil	Coconut oil
Flaxseed oil **	Canola oil	Cotton seed oil
		Animal fat shortening
		Lard and beef fat

* Ghee (clarified butter) can be prepared by gently warming the butter and skimming off the top layer of "white fats" rich in saturated and polyunsaturated fats and milk proteins; the latter seems to improve the tolerance of ghee for many individuals who are sensitive to milk proteins.

** Flaxseed oil is an excellent source of omega-3 and omega-6 oils. Cold pressed flaxseed oil should be purchased in dark bottles and should be kept refrigerated with the cap tightly closed. Three 200 mg capsules of vitamin E added to the bottle of flaxseed oil are very effective in preventing undesirable oxidation of flaxseed oil.

Supplemental oils:

Evening primrose oil   Black currant oil   Borage oil

Aging-Oxidant oils:

Margarine*   Vegetable shortening   Animal fat shortening
Cholesterol-free fatty Foods**

   * Margarine contain up to 35% of fats as trans fatty acids which cannot be utilized by human tissues. Trans fatty acids raise the blood levels of LDL ("bad") cholesterol and lower blood levels of HDL ("good") cholesterol.

   ** Cholesterol-free fats are rendered "cholesterol-free" through chemical processes that introduce trans fatty acids and toxic cyclic compounds into these fats. Trans fatty acids and toxic cyclic fatty compounds cannot be metabolized by the body and, quite literally, clog up the molecular wheels of fat metabolism in the body. The immune system resents this onslaught of toxic molecules and mounts an immune response by making antibodies specifically directed against these toxic compounds. These antibodies try to capture these toxic compounds by making complexes with them and clear them, but have a limited capacity for it. With passing years, denatured and toxic fats in supermarket foods prove to be too large a burden for the immune system to bear. Complexes formed of toxic fats and antibodies accumulate within the lining of the blood vessels, and plaque begin to form. Research also shows how trans fatty acids raise LDL cholesterol and lower HDL cholesterol, changes which further impair normal cholesterol metabolism (N Eng J Med 323:439; 1990). I discuss this important subject in depth in my monograph *Choua, Cholesterol Cats and Chelation.*

Carbohydrates

Choice One	Choice Two	Choice Three
Brown rice	Rye#	Wheat#
Barley	Buckwheat	Corn
Wild rice	Oats#	White rice
Amaranth	Potato	
Millet	Barley#	
Artichoke	Yam	
Quinoa, Tapioca, milo		
Soy products (Tofu, Tampeh)		
Spelt, Kamut and Teff*		
Nuts and seeds** and others***		

Gluten-sensitive persons need to avoid or restrict wheat, rye, oat and barley — grains that contain "free gluten"; other grains such as amaranth, buckwheat, quinoa, milo, teff, rice and corn contain small amounts of "bound gluten" that, in general, do not cause food incompatibility reactions in gluten-sensitive persons. * Spelt and Kumat are two types of ancient wheats that appear to be antigenically distinct enough from the common wheat to be tolerated well by individuals who suffer from wheat incompatibility. These are usually grown without pesticides. Spelt has a strong hull that protects its kernel. Teff, an Ethiopian staple, is a highly nutritious grain that contains more than ten times as much calcium as wheat and barley.
** Sunflower seeds, sesame seeds, pumpkin seeds, melon seeds, watermelon seeds, soy nuts (actually a grain), cashew nuts, macadamia nuts, pine nuts, brazil nuts, chestnut, pecans, and litchi nuts. *Peanuts and walnuts are common causes of allergic reactions and should be eaten infrequently.*
*** Malanga, yuca, sesame meal, sunflower meal, breadfruit, lotus root, agar. Beans: black beans, pink beans, white beans, hokaido beans and others.

Comment

Wheat and corn are excellent sources of proteins and carbohydrates.

However these grains are eaten every day by many people. People with allergic genes generally become allergic to the foods that they eat most frequently. This explains why these grains rank high among the list of allergenic foods. White rice is included here because it has been literally stripped of all its nutrients. Another important reason behind my choices among grain is that wholesome life-span nutrition requires diversity. Addiction to these grains (food allergy and food addiction are the two sides of the same coin) is often the primary reason of lack for diversity in nutrition for many people.

Proteins

Choice One

Hunted Fish*
Lentils
Beans**
Duck, quail
Venison, elk
Antelope
Rabbit, pheasant
Goat, sheep, wild buffalo
Guinea hen, muscovy duck
Amino acid, peptide and protein formulas****
Whole grains
Spirolina plankton

Choice Two

Chicken
Turkey
Shellfish
Cornish hen
Egg***

Choice Three

Beef
Veal
Cultured fish
Pork

Comment

* Sea Bass, Red Snapper, Atlantic Paddock and Rock Fish are excellent low-fat fish (A 3 1/2-ounce portion of each of sea bass and chinook salmon contains 595 and 1,355 mg of Omega-3; the respective numbers for total fat are 3 and 10 grams). Other good choices are catfish, cod, grouper, halibut, haddock, herring, mackerel, mahi, and pike. Cultured fish are increasingly raised in fisheries that use large amounts of fungicides and antibiotics to increase the fish yield. Beef and egg rank high among the causes of food allergy.

** Beans such as grains can be budded (sprouted) to enhance their nutritional value. Budding increases the vitamin B complex levels by many folds and also has the effect of predigesting these foods. Zuki and Mung beans are especially good for this purpose.

*** Egg is an excellent source of high-grade proteins and lecithin (the "good" fat that facilitates metabolism of fat and prevents fat buildup in the liver and other body tissues). However, as I indicated earlier, the frequency of egg allergy in the general population is quite high.

**** We need proteins for their amino acids. We need amino acids as building blocks for tissue proteins, hormones and neurotransmitters. As a source of energy, I regard them as "time-release energy molecules." Amino acids are also the premium intelligence molecules of the body. Properly formulated amino acid and peptide products prepared from natural proteins by partial hydrolysis (predigestion) are excellent sources of these nutrients. Many of the popular brand protein drinks carry 50 to 90% calories as carbohydrates. I do not recommend such products. Good amino acid, peptide and protein formulas should have as much as 90% calories as these nutrients.

The life span advantages of amino acids are too numerous to be enumerated here. I discuss elsewhere in this volume the health hazards of sugar. Sugar is a much bigger culprit than fat in the cause of degenerative and immune disorder. In this context, well-formulated amino acid, peptide (small chains of amino acids) and protein products, when taken with vegetable and fruity juices or with dilute soy or rice milk, make an excellent breakfast. Indeed, my own breakfast 3 to 4 days a week is composed of an amino acid and protein formula mixed with one of the above fluids. I do not need any coffee or tea. It sustains me till my lunch. I use three formulas made from different sources of protein to balance the intake of various amino acids contained in them. I recommend such well-formulated products to my patients, especially those who suffer from molecular roller coasters or experience rapid hypoglycemic-hyperglycemic shifts. *It is imperative, however, that amino acid, peptide and protein drinks be used under the general supervision of a knowledgeable professional.*

Low-Fat Meats

There are some well-touted methods for commercially producing "lean meats" by feeding the livestock different types of feeds. In recent years, there have also been attempts to produce "better meats" by administering growth hormone to cattle. These *clever* ways of altering the natural order of things are of no interest to people interested in nutrition for the life span. I do not recommend these meats.

There are some other time-honored methods for cooking meats to significantly lower their fat (and cholesterol) content. Perhaps the oldest and the best-known method is the method of preparing *Yekhani* (a type of fat-free broth) from the meat, and then cooking the meat with yekhani. These methods are extremely useful in lowering the saturated fats and cholesterol content of different types of meats. I strongly recommend them.

An excellent method for successfully defatting meats rich in saturated fats was recently described. In this method:

1.   Ground meats are partially cooked in olive oil or other suitable vegetable oils.
2.   Meats are next rinsed with boiling water to extract fats and cholesterol.
3.   Broth is prepared by separating fats from the water used for rinsing meat.
4.   Meats are cooked to completion with the fat-free broth obtained from the water used for rinsing (restoring the flavor and minerals in the meat).
5.   Meats are now ready to be used in meat loaf, chili, soups, sauces, spaghetti and other dishes.

Saturated fats and cholesterol dissolve in vegetable oils only to a limited degree (only about one-half teaspoonful of meat fats dissolves in 3 ounces of vegetable oils at room temperature). However, at cooking temperatures, 5 to 10 times as much cholesterol will dissolve in the same volume of oil. In an extensive series of experiments, large quantities of saturated fats (from 72 to 87 %) were removed from beef and pork by the above method (N. Eng. J. Med 324:73; 1991).

"Enriched" Cereals Are Poor Foods

Our food industry gives unique meanings to the word "enriched." During the processing of "enriching" our cereals and grains, it strips our foods of several valuable nutrients and then adds four items back. That earns for them, these merchants of our food industry, the right to label their food products as "enriched." Specifically, the process of enrichment adds three vitamins (thiamin, niacin, and riboflavin) and one mineral (iron). Now let us consider what it takes out: calcium, magnesium, manganese, potassium, phosphorus, zinc, vitamin B-6 and vitamin E. Such enrichment we can do without.

Aging-Oxidant Meats

Deli meats and other highly salted, highly processed and highly spices meats are obviously not good food choices.

Vegetables

Choice One	Choice Two
Daikon	Romaine lettuce
Burdock	Boston lettuce
Red radish	Iceberg lettuce
Squashes *	Spinach
Chinese cabbage	Onion
Turnips	Carrot
Green beans	Tomato
Shiitake mushrooms	Red peppers
Lotus root	Green peppers
Turnips	Yam
Green Beans	Egg plant
Green leafy vegetables **	
Others ***	
Ginger	

* Squashes: acorn, buttercup, butternut, hokaido, hubbard, spaghetti, star, yellow summer, zucchini.
** Lettuce substitutes: green tops of beets, carrot, collard, daikon, kale, mustard, red radish, spinach and turnip.
*** artichoke, asparagus, beets, brussel sprouts, broccoli, bok choy, cabbage, cauliflower, celery, cucumber, escarole, garlic, ginger, parsnip, peas, plantain, rutabagas, sauerkraut, scallions, shiitake mushroom, water chestnut.

Lettuce is in the same family as ragweed, which is among the most allergenic weeds in the United States. There is a high degree of cross reactivity between lettuce and ragweed. For this reason I recommend people with food and hay-fever type allergy to cut down on lettuce and use lettuce substitutes given above.

Vegetables for use as condiments:

Chives   dandelion   Endives

Garlic	Ginger	Nori
Parsley	Scallions	

All of the above condiments may be considered Choice One foods except when sensitivity to these foods exists.

Wild Vegetables

Wild burdock	Dandelion	Ferns*
Horsetail	Lamb quarter	Milkweed
Mugwort	Weeds*	

* Knotweed, Pigweed, Thistle

All wild vegetables are considered Choice One foods. Wild vegetables are especially rich in minerals and vitamins. For instance, weight for weight dandelion contains about 8 times as much calcium as milk.

Sea Vegetables

Sea vegetables (algae, grasses and other edible plants) have been used by almost all coastal cultures in different parts of the world. The recognized health benefits include functional restoration of stomach, bowel, kidneys, brain, cardiovascular system and skin. As for wild vegetables, all sea vegetables are considered Choice One vegetables.

Kombu	Wakame	Hiziki
Nori	Agar	Mekabu
Dulse		

Fruits

Choice One	Choice Two	Choice Three
Peach	Lemon & Lime	Orange
Pear	Fig	Pineapple
Cherries	Raisins	Coconut
Berries*	Melon	Strawberries
Avocado	Watermelon	Grapes
Plum	Kiwi	Honeydew
Apricot	Grapefruit	Mangoes
Papaya	Cantaloupe	Dates
Guava	Plum	Polished fruits#
Persimmon	Banana	
Pomegranate		
Rhubarb		
Prune		
Organic Apples#		

The fruits in the third category are included there for reasons of their high fructose content, acidity and the potential to cause allergy. Fruits should be eaten fresh in season. Avoid completely canned fruit. Depleted of their life-sustaining enzymes and laced with sugar, canned fruits in reality are canned candy.

*   Blueberries, Blackberries, Cranberries and Raspberries.

The issue of pesticide and fungicide residue over fruits and vegetables is an important issue. All fruits and vegetables should be thoroughly washed to eliminate, or at least reduce, such residues. Polished fruits present a more complex problem. Organically grown unpolished apples are among the first choice group for their long-established empirical nutritional value. I list apples treated with pesticides and polished to improve their looks for equally obvious reasons. I strongly recommend the following simple experiment to understand the nature of the problems caused by pesticides and waxing the apple skin. Put a healthy-looking, well-polished apple in a pot, cover it with hot water for two minutes, shake the pot for a minute or

so, take the apple out and let it dry. Now observe the surface of the water in the pot for wax globules and the apple skin for its true color and texture. Almost all pesticides are fat-soluble. Multiple applications of wax to the apple skin has the effect of embedding the pesticides deep in the layers of wax. Simple washing of apples creates an illusion of removing the wax and the pesticides blended in it. The first time I did this simple experiment I was horrified to see the results.

Life-Span and Aging-Oxidant Desserts

Life-Span Desserts

The critical issues in desserts from a life span perspectives are:

* Use of fruits juices versus sugar as sweetener
* Use of natural food sweeteners such as liquorice, carob, cinnamon, molasses, Pilon Cillo and honey.
* Use of other sweeteners such as food grain glycerine and herbs like Stevia and Tree Sweet.
* Occasional use of artificial sweeteners such as Aspartame and saccharine except for people with chemical sensitivity to these items.

Sugar: A Nutritional Villain

Sugar is an antinutrient. Ideally all desserts should be prepared with fruit juices or natural sweeteners such as honey and stevia. Fruits contain fructose, which is metabolized at a slower rate than glucose in sugar. More importantly, fruit juices are very rich sources of mineral cofactors and some digestive enzymes. Sugar, of course, is totally devoid of any nutritional merit and is one of the principal nutritional villains.

Preparing desserts with natural sweeteners within reason is an acceptable practice for those who can be comfortable with restraints implicit in this practice. Some good choices include rice syrup, almond syrup, maple syrup, persimmon, honey and carob. For others, such desserts may be combined at times with those prepared with aspartame and saccharine. Similarly, diet sodas with aspartame are allowed within reason.

Aging-Oxidant Desserts

| Cakes | Candy | Caramel |
| Chocolate | Cookies | Creams |

My editor read the draft of this chapter and wrote the following note on the border, "You're taking all the fun out of life! No more pie a'lamode?!" Yes! That's way the way it sounds to the beginner. Life span nutrition, I wrote earlier, is not about denial of dieting or euphoria of eating. However, it does take some time before a metabolism burdened with the massive overload of oxidized and denatured supermarket foods begins to recover and gives a resounding testimony to the validity of the principles and practice of life span nutrition.

There are many hidden sources of sugar in American diet. For instance, ketchup is rich in sugar. Moist dates are moist due to added syrup and contain much more sugar than loose dates. Fruits are often unrecognized but rich sources of sugar.

Keeping these foods in the house for the company should be resisted at all times. Sugar craving is caused by salt, sugar and molecular roller coasters (discussed in the chapter On Limbic Eating). Serious difficulties with sugar craving usually require skillful professional management. This problem cannot be addressed by keeping desserts in the house for company. Company can get their fix of aging-oxidant foods elsewhere.

Snacks

Snacks are best avoided. Regular meals at regular times is the best strategy for good health for the life span. It is sadly ironic that we *train* our children to demand snacks while we as adults struggle to unlearn this awful habit. Most commonly eaten snacks are neat packages of highly oxidized foods, wonderful prescriptions for degenerative and immune disorders and for premature aging. If habit makes complete avoidance of snacks difficult in the beginning or when the rush of metabolic roller coasters is insufferable, the following snacks may be eaten.

Sunflower Seeds	Pumpkin Seeds	Sesame Seeds
Popped Amaranth	Popcorn*	Popped millet
Sprouted Grains*	Buckwheat	Vegetables

* A fascinating phenomenon in the human experience for me is this: We see somethings almost every day but their profound

significance escapes us for years until some *limbic moment* brings home the truth. I love to walk in woods around our house in Blairstown. How often have I seen seeds germinate? How often have seen little twigs raising their proud heads from the dirt in springtime? I often stop in my walks to observe these beginnings of life. These tiny occurrences of growth symbolize new beginnings, new hopes, new lives. What biochemistry in nature sustains such occurrences? This question never crossed my mind during years of walking in the woods. In the days I worked on this chapter, a twig appeared before me during my limbic run one morning. Suddenly, there was a new sense of energy about this twig which I had never known before. In the shower after the run, the question of biochemistry sustaining that energy arose in my mind.

When the seeds germinate, the amount of some vitamins in them rises steeply, by some estimates as much as sixty-fold. This phenomenon is most pronounced for members of vitamin B complex. Why? Because the needs for life-giving enzymes in budding seeds increase sharply. What are B vitamins but life-giving enzymes. So that's it! I shook with excitement as I realized how intuitive people in all cultures and in all parts of the world learned the value of sprouting seeds and grains before eating them.

SUGAR BLUES, BETA BLOCKER BLUES
AND BLOATING BLUES

Fruits in general are excellent life span foods. Fruits are rich in vitamins and minerals, and of course carry live enzymes.

Fructose is metabolized by the tissues at a slower rate than is glucose. Nevertheless, sugar content of fruits is an important issue in life span nutrition. For many people with increased sensitivity to sugars, even fruits cause sugar blues.

In the subsequent chapter On Limbic Eating, I discuss how increased oxidative molecular injury and immune disorders put substantial stresses on the thyroid, pancreas and adrenal glands. This is the main reason why people with these disorders frequently suffer from hypothyroidism (underactive thyroid gland), hypoglycemia and chronic stress syndrome. It is not uncommon for me to see patients who suffer from these disorders and who react poorly to large quantities of fructose consumed with fruits.

Two other important points may be made in our discussion of sugar blues and fruits: the impact of beta blocker drugs and the altered states of bowel ecology on sugar blues. Beta blockers, as is implied in their name, block beta receptors, and are used to "block" the adrenergic overdrive. Beta blockers not only block this overdrive (a euphemism for molecular hyper-vigilance of chronic stress syndrome), they also cause undue tiredness, mood disorders and depression, the so-called beta blocker blues. Since stress is a dominant part of the clinical picture of most chronic disorders, and since we physicians only know how to pay lip service to "stress reduction," we find beta blocker drugs a godsend. Those of us who practice drug medicine dole out beta blocker prescriptions as pediatricians dispense candy to children during their office visits with them. This is how the trouble begins: I see many sugar-sensitive patients who can tolerate fructose in fruits but react poorly when they take beta blockers drugs. Beta blocker drugs in this setting turn some life span fruits into aging-oxidant fruits.

A similar situation is often observed in patients with altered bowel ecology states. Abdominal bloating and flatulence are major clinical problems when the internal ecology of the bowel is disturbed. Many sugar-sensitive individuals can cope with fructose load and eat fruits with many nutritional benefits when the internal ecology of the bowel is normal. However, the concurrent intake of beta-blockers and fruits rich in fructose in the presence of altered states of bowel ecology often leads to sugar roller coasters and more intense abdominal symptoms. Again, an altered state of bowel ecology can turn life span fruits into aging-oxidant foods. Some fruits are very effective in regulating bowel transit time. Apples are high in pectin and soluble fiber. Peaches, pears and plums are among fruits that add roughage to the bowel. Prunes increase the bowel transit time and are quite well known for what they do.

HOW DO AMINO ACIDS WORK?

Amino acids are used by our tissues in countless ways. Protein predigestion vastly improves their rate of absorption and facilitates their utilization in the tissues. The more predigested are the proteins in a given formula, the more hypoallergenic it is. A full discussion of the role of amino acids in health preservation is outside the scope of this volume. I include some brief comments for general interest of the reader.

I begin with taurine, my favorite for many reasons. Taurine is a major antioxidant, and plays a critical role in preserving the integrity of plasma membrane, the true interface between internal order and external disorder for the cell. Taurine helps in the maintenance of the membrane potential in the muscle and nerve cell, hence its role in regulation of heart rhythm, neurotransmitter functions and body temperature. Taurine stabilizes calcium and potassium in cell membranes of heart and brain cells in stressful physiologic and pathologic states. Taurine is structurally similar to both choline and GABA, and has been reported to be beneficial in both experimental and clinical epilepsy. Taurine can be formed in gut by bacterial enzymes (bacterial enzymes also serve as life span enzymes for humans). J. Awapara wrote in *Taurine* "... taurine exists uncombined and distributed throughout the animal kingdom in a manner almost unparalleled by any other small organic molecule." (page 19, Raven Press New York 1976). Nature is not wasteful, and from a purely teleological standpoint, one can consider taurine distribution in tissues by itself a strong evidence for its functional universality. I use taurine as a nutrient supplement liberally for my patients with accelerated oxidative molecular injury who present with chronic fatigue and indolent immune disorders.

Some amino acids such as carnitine, ornithine and arginine are valuable for supporting muscle energy metabolism. Carnitine completes one of the main steps in fat breakdown. Some studies show evidence that lack of carnitine can lead to excessive fat accumulation in tissues. I find carnitine of considerable clinical value in people with low general energy level and those who suffer from chronic fatigue. As we grow old, the level of growth hormone in tissues decline. Lowered levels of growth hormone are considered to be related to aging changes seen in people. Some studies show that arginine and ornithine can stimulate the production of growth hormone, and in this indirect way, serve as life span molecules. These amino acids also play key roles in detoxification processes in the liver.

Methionine, another important amino acid, serves as a major lipotropic factor and facilitates fat metabolism in the liver. It also serves as precursor of cystine and cysteine, and together these three amino acids serve as a major sulfur-containing (sulfhydryl) antioxidant system of the body.

Some amino acids such as tyrosine and tryptophane are very useful for improving neurotransmitter functions. It is most unfortunate that tryptophane has been taken off the market because some batches prepared by one manufacturer were contaminated with a toxin. Now tryptophane is unavailable to hundred of thousands of people with depression and anxiety who used to take tryptophane to ameliorate their suffering and avoid serious toxic effects of drugs which they are now forced to take. It is somewhat like government taking bananas off nation's markets just because some shipments from one city in South America were contaminated. Such is the official wisdom! Such is the helplessness of those who suffer.

Histidine is converted into histamine which is an important mediator molecule of inflammatory response and repair reaction. I use it in my "nutrient anti-histaminic" formula. Glycine and amino-butyric acid are inhibitory neurotransmitter that prevent abnormal firing of nerve cells. Aspartic acid is involved in detoxification reactions in the liver, facilitates disposal of ammonia, and is of value in chronic fatigue and muscle pain. Alanine and proline are used in the body for synthesis of pantothenic acid and collagen respectively. Leucine, along with glutamine, is useful for stabilizing blood glucose levels. Glycine, glutamic acid and lysine (when used in combination with saw palmetto, zinc and manganese) is effective in up to two-thirds of people with enlarged prostate. Valine is some general stimulatory effects, but its effects have not been studied well. It is better not to use it as a single agent, especially for people with heart disease.

In May 1992, at the conference of the American College for Advancement in Medicine, I had the great honor of presenting the 1992 Achievement Award of the College to Linus Pauling. Pauling, the only living person to receive two unshared Nobel prizes, advised us to use lysine along with vitamin C for prevention and treatment of heart disease. His told us of his intuitive insight into the presence of lysine in certain molecules that normally preserve the health of connective tissue in arteries. Of course, we physicians in general detest such intuitive recommendations that have not been proven with our *blessed* double-blind cross-over research model. As for me, I treasure insights of my patients and all others who have notions of helping people live longer, healthier and happier. No one ranks higher than Linus Pauling when it comes to that. I am wary, I might add, of the great intuitive insights of physician-speakers on the payroll of our drug companies and who regularly extol the virtues of drugs made by their payors.

Returning to the subject of proteins, good sources of proteins are also good sources of essential oils belonging to Omega-3 (predominantly of marine source) and Omega-6 (predominantly of plant source) types. There is strong circumstantial evidence that the great increase in degenerative disorders that has accompanied "great advances" in food technology in this country is causally related to an increase in toxic fat intake and a decrease in the Omega-3:Omega-6 ratio. An excellent solution to this problem is to make fish a regular source of protein in the weekly nutritional plan.

Minerals

Life Span Minerals and Aging-Oxidant Minerals

Life span minerals sustain life; aging-oxidant minerals cause premature aging.

Examples of life span minerals are iron, calcium, sodium, potassium, magnesium, zinc, selenium, molybdenum, chromium, copper, cobalt, boron and others. Examples of aging oxidant minerals are lead, mercury, aluminum, tin, cadmium, gold and others.

Our science and technology have brought forth many benefits for us. We recognize them fully. Our science and technology have also wreaked havoc on our ecology. We do not fully recognize this. Perhaps nowhere is the damage caused by technology to our ecology more damaging or pervasive than in the changes caused in the mineral content of our water, food and tissues. We are being systematically depleted of life span minerals as we are being overloaded with aging oxidant minerals.

Minerals are the life-blood of enzymes.

Enzymes sustain life by generating energy. Enzyme assemble molecules for building tissues. Enzymes split and re-shape molecules for remodeling tissues. Enzymes add molecules up for storing energy. Enzymes slice molecules to release energy for life functions. Enzymes are proteins that the body can freely produce. Minerals, by contrast, must be obtained from the food. Mineral deficiencies occur frequently when sufficient minerals are not present in food or are not absorbed.

Early symptoms of mineral deficiency are in reality symptoms of enzyme insufficiency.

The subject of mineral deficiencies is a misunderstood subject. How do mineral deficiencies put our health in jeopardy? In scientific jargon, minerals are considered cofactors for enzymes. It means the enzymes depend upon minerals for their function. In mineral deficiency states, the enzymes become sluggish or paralyzed, enzyme detoxification systems are impaired, and a state of "absence of health" develops. This is the beginning of many chronic disorders. Since the early clinical symptoms of mineral deficiency actually appear as enzymatic dysfunctions, they often go unrecognized. A good example of this is the pervasive magnesium deficiency among Americans. If not reversed, this state of absence of health evolves into a full expression of clinical disease.

Pro-oxidant Minerals

Three essential minerals stand out in this special category: iron, copper and iodine. All three serve as cofactors for oxygen and facilitate oxidation of many molecules. The deficiency states of all three cause well-recognized disorders (anemia for iron, hypothyroidism for iodine and anemia for copper). The overload of all three causes many enzymatic dysfunctions. Thus, supplementation for these minerals should always be carefully supervised by a professional.

A practical point of considerable importance is that when these three minerals are taken as supplements, they should be taken separately from vitamin supplements, essential fatty acid and amino acid supplements. Most mineral supplements can be taken at night, while others can be taken in the morning.

Sodium: A Life Span Mineral Turned Aging-Oxidant Mineral

Sodium is an essential mineral for human metabolism. It has become an aging-oxidant mineral. It is an excellent example of how some life span molecules have been turned into aging oxidative molecules by standard American foods.

There is such an excess of table salt (sodium chloride) in our common foods that salt has become one of the major risk factors for hypertension (high blood pressure), heart disease, stroke and kidney disease. See the Appendix for the sodium contents of some commonly eaten foods.

Excess sodium is a major cause of sugar craving.

Among the prevalent adverse effects of excess of salt in

food are sugar craving, water retention, PMS syndrome, arthralgia (stiff and painful joints), mental confusion, short attention span and inexplicable mood swings. Following are some practical suggestions for reducing the load of this life span mineral turned aging-oxidant mineral.

COMMON SOURCES OF SALT LOADING

1. Deli foods are rich in salt, rich in oxidized fats, rich in calories and poor in nutrients and in common sense.
2. Garlic salt, celery salt and bouillon cubes contain large amounts of salt.
3. Canned foods are often laced with salt.
4. Canned vegetable juices (a can of salted V8 has about 600 mg of sodium, unsalted V 8 has only a few mg). Commercial salad dressings, sauces, soups and chutneys.

Creative Seasoning Without Table Salt

Examples: Use low-salt products. Tabasco brand pepper sauce has only 2.5 mg of sodium per average serving. Substitute lime, lemon or grapefruit juices for salted vinegar and wines in marinades. Order oil and vinegar separately for mixing your own low-salt dressing. Sprinkle basil, dill or oregano on corn.

Cooking With Less Salt, Sugar and Fat
(and more flavor, texture and taste)

1. Flavor hot dishes with spices to reduce the need for salt and fat. Example: Cajun cooking.
2. Flavor deserts with extracts: vanilla, almond butter, cashew butter to reduce the need for salt, sugar and fats.
3. Flavor dishes with wine or sherry to reduce need for salt, butter and creams for soup.
4. Enhance texture and taste of soups with French bread, beans, carrots and pureed potatoes.
5. Enhance texture and taste of foods with sunflower, sesame and poppy seeds.
6. Enhance taste of chicken and fish with mandarin, pineapple, papaya, mango and other fruits.
7. Enhance taste of hard cereals with fruit butters, cinnamon or similar ingredients.
8. Enhance taste of hot dishes with natural herbs and use less salt and fats.
9. Thickening items: agar, kuzu, arrowroot, brown rice flower, barley grits and tofu.
10. Special items for preparing sauces for cooking: miso, soy sauce, tahini, kuzu.

Sea salt is rich in many trace minerals and accentuates food with much less sodium load than the common table salt. Prepare your own seasonings and broth with small quantities of sea salt. Potassium salt is recommended as a substitute for table salt on an occasional basis. It does not carry the risk of sodium overload, and it provides potassium, which is often deficient in the standard American diet.

TOXIC METALS

The incidence of heavy toxic metal overload in human tissues is rising at an enormous rate. My clinical work with patients with chronic fatigue has convinced me that this is a major emerging threat to human biology. I test these individuals for aluminum, mercury, lead, cadmium and arsenic. Nearly one-third of my patients show elevated blood levels of one or more of these metals. The sources of these toxic metals are not always clear to me. Aluminum is present in most antacids and deodorants. Aluminum cookware is another recognizable source. It is my strong sense that the primary source of toxic metals is our water supply. Acid rains increase the soil acidity and leach metals out of it. These toxic metals are potent poisons for life span enzymes. The clinical improvement of people with chronic fatigue is markedly slowed down unless toxic metals are chelated out of their bodies.

My friend, Stephen Davies, M.D., one of the eminent British nutritionist-physicians presented frightening data at the spring 1992 meeting of the American College for Advancement in Medicine held in Dallas. He reported data gathered with his studies of over 15,000 individuals conducted over several years. These data clearly documented what people have known intuitively: The body burden of toxic metals is steadily rising in human tissues. The observed increase in the body burden of toxic minerals correlates directly with the increasing age of subjects studied.

Dead bodies are the only proof some professional accept for heavy metal toxicity.

We physicians have some understanding of the acute toxicity of heavy metals. In general, our knowledge of the slow and sustained molecular injury caused by progressive accumulation of toxic metals in our tissues is fragmentary. Sometimes this lack of knowledge leads to silly (and amusing) debates among physicians. Once a physician employed by one of the State Departments of Health called me about one of my patients who was found to have high blood mercury levels. She repeatedly asked me if the patient salivated excessively. I told her the patient did not. This disturbed her to no end. She could not understand why I wanted to chelate mercury out of her body when one of the classical signs of mercury toxicity (excessive salivation) was not present. Some old medical texts hold that excessive salivation is an essential sign of mercury toxicity. The concept of ill effects of cumulative body burdens of toxic metals is hard for some professionals to understand. Dead bodies, it seems to me, is the proof many of my colleagues insist upon for heavy metal toxicity.

VEGETABLE AND FRUIT JUICES

I cannot overstate the case for investing in a juicer. Also,

I cannot overstate the case for investing a few minutes in preparing fresh vegetable juice. Chlorophyll, I wrote early, is what turns solar energy into chemical bond energy for the food chain in nature. Vegetables are the best sources of chlorophyll. Vegetables are the best source of minerals. And, of course, fresh vegetables are the best source of life span enzymes. I discuss this subject further in the chapter On Limbic Eating.

THE MERCHANTS OF "ENRICHED" FOODS

The profit for our wealthy cholesterol and cereal industries are in the sales of the so-called cholesterol-lowering drugs and fiber-rich "enriched" cereals. Their "enlightened" marketing strategies call for emphasis on disease prevention. So what do they do? They pepper their advertisements with some neat advice about consuming fiber to lower cholesterol. They, and physicians on their payroll, never tell us that foods with high fiber content contain large amounts of phytates that block absorption of essential minerals such as calcium, magnesium and others. I am not sure of the benefits of lowering blood cholesterol levels a few points with large amounts of fiber that interfere with absorption of calcium, magnesium and many other essential minerals.

In my monograph, *Choua, Cholesterol Cats and Chelation,* I describe how the blood cholesterol level only serves as a marker of heart disease, a poor one at that except for a small number of people with genetic factors which drastically raise blood cholesterol levels. This means that the factors which cause heart disease also raise blood cholesterol levels. It appears highly doubtful to me that blood cholesterol level will ever prove to be a risk factor for heart disease except in a small number of people with hereditary lipid disorders. This means that simply lowering cholesterol will not protect us from heart disease, just as lowering the blood level of CEA (a marker of colon cancer) will not prevent death from colon cancer.

While we are just beginning to recognize our error in mindlessly blaming the natural, un-oxidized cholesterol molecule for everything, we have no doubt about the dangers of essential mineral deficiencies. The advertisements of cereal companies tell us about their cereals enriched with iron, iodine and thiamine. What they do not tell us is that their "enrichment" process robs the cereals of calcium, magnesium, manganese, potassium, phosphorus, zinc and several vitamins and life span enzymes. The advertisements of the merchants of drugs tell us all about how their drugs lower blood cholesterol levels but do not tell us how their drugs cripple enzymes that normally metabolize cholesterol. The advertisements of the fiber industry are silent on how fiber interferes with essential mineral absorption. I wonder why none of our legislators ever thought of a "the *whole* truth in advertising" bill.

FOODS AS REMEDIES

The use of foods as healing substances is a lost art. Foods have been successfully used for non-life-threatening conditions for centuries. Their use is, of course, most beneficial when in the hands of physicians who can separate serious diseases from common maladies. It is unfortunate how our infatuation with drugs has made us physicians turn our backs to all uses of foods as remedies. Food are non-toxic and completely free of any side effects.

It's not news that eating certain foods helps prevent cancer; the big question is why? Now researchers believe they are closing in on some answers. .... a band of chemists, biochemists, and molecular biologists has started to map out the specific compounds in foods that give them their anticancer properties, and they are beginning to discover how these chemicals disrupt the molecular pathways that lead to cancer.

Science 257:1349; 1992

Science fills the gaps created by intuition. This happens in all branches of scientific inquiry, and is often a very slow process. Intuition leaps where science must be cautious and painstaking. The ancients were astute observers of human nutrition and health, and they left behind for us an enormous legacy of intuitive wisdom. They made many empirical observation about the healthful effects of certain foods. We are just beginning to understand the scientific basis of some of these observations. A full treatment of this subject is outside the scope of this book. As a matter of some general interest for the reader, I cite two examples of soybean and broccoli.

No food fascinates me more than soybean when I reflect upon empirical observations — and intuitive insights — of the ancients about this grain. In the section dealing with life span enzymes, I describe how each major culture of the Far East developed its own version of predigested soybean dishes as their staple foods. Now let us consider what is in soybean and what it can do for human cells.

Soybeans contains large quantities of phospholipids and lecithin that are essential for the structural and functional integrity of cell membranes and the plasma membranes of organelles within the cells. Cell membranes, I wrote earlier separate an internal order of the cell from an external disorder. Phospolipids are electrically charged molecules and play critical roles in cellular intelligence systems. These lipids also provide raw materials for the synthesis of prostaglandins, leukotrienes and some other molecules that defend cell innards against noxious agents that surround cells. These essential fats improves memory and mental functions, facilitates fat metabolism, prevents plaque formation in the heart and arteries, protects liver from cirrhosis, and is essential for growth of children. For sometime now, my research associate, Gary Viole, and I have been studying the enormous value of soybean phospholipids as agents that promote healing of open wounds and as antiviral agents.

When the healthful phospholipids are oxidized and denatured, the immune system recognizes them as such and tries to rid the body of them by making antibodies against them. Antiphospholipid antibodies so formed, in their confusion of purpose, destroy blood platelets, cause clot formation within blood vessels and lead to a host of clinical syndromes. Indeed, so wide is the array of such clinical conditions that the term antiphospholipid antibody syndrome has been proposed as a unifying concept (*Br J Rhuematol* 26:324; 1987). Soybeans contain 3 isoflavones, substances that break down toxins and reduce risk of cancer.

Is it a pure coincidence that soybean was recognized as an especially healthful food by the ancients and as a an especially rich source of essential phospholipids and other healthy fats by modern chemistry? The ancients didn't know chemistry of soybean, at least in the way we know it. What led the ancients to their great intuitive insights about soybean? An interesting questions!

Some years ago, Japanese researchers reported studies that suggested soybean may be a culprit in the high incidence of cancer in Japan. Japanese are meticulous investigators and one does not lightly challenge their research methods or conclusions. Still, I felt considerable difficulty in accepting their viewpoint. My reason: The study conclusions seem to fly in the face of the many empirical observations about soybean made by the ancient. Specifically, how could so may different peoples of the Far East have made such a bad mistake, and for so many thousands of years. How could they have missed the link between soybean and cancer if any did exist? I wondered about the Japanese report and kept my reservation about its validity.

Nothing could be further from the truth, says Michael Pariza, a food researcher at the University of Wisconsin, Madison. Pariza discovered that soybean actually inhibits stomach cancer in mice, and recently he has isolated an ingredient that appears to be responsible. It is called HEMF (for 4-hydroxy-2-ethyl-5-methyl-3 (2H)-furanone and it is, Pariza says, what gives soy sauce its distinctive flavor.

Science 257:1349; 1992

Broccoli restores bowel ecology; strengthens the immune system; contains organosulfer compounds, indole carbinol (which breaks down estrogen) and beta carotene which is an important anti-oxidant. All of these substances have proven anticancer activities. Cabbage, cauliflower are brussels sprouts are cousin cruciferous vegetables of broccoli that share with it cancer-preventing agents. Specifically, anethole trithione is one specific sulfer-containing natural compound isolated from broccoli that has been shown to prevent colon cancer in rats.

I include below a list of ten of my favorite foods with their medicinal benefits. This is followed by some other selected foods with their empirical therapeutic uses which have been recorded over the centuries.

TEN FOODS OF SPECIAL HEALTHFUL EFFECTS

Soybean and Broccoli. Burdock has long established

empirical value in improving digestive and absorptive functions in the stomach and bowel, facilitates bowel transit time, restores bowel ecology state. **Celery** contains heart-friendly phthalate, and is helpful in lowering high blood pressure and normalizing blood lipids. Celery is also beneficial for joint symptoms and for related disorders such as bursitis and fibrositis. **Daikon** has long-established empirical value in maintaining a healthy bowel ecology. See the note for burdock. **Flaxseed** contains linolenic acid, an essential fatty acid, which reduces the formation of hormone-like substances called prostaglandins of PG-2 series. These prostaglandins induce inflammatory response in lungs (asthma), joints (arthritis), skin (psoriasis) and other body organs. Prostaglandins may also contribute to development of tumors. Flaxseed is a cereal grain that Europeans and Canadians consume in large quantities in their cereals and breads. **Garlic** contains allicin and some other sulfur compounds that restore bowel ecology, prevent yeast overgrowth, thin blood, prevent platelet clumping, appear to act as an anti-inflammatory agent and antibacterial agent and reduce the risk of cancer.

Ginger contains natural alkaloids that precipitate out (and render harmless) most environmental pollutants in the drinking water. (see note about ginger root water in the beverage section of this chapter). Long-established empirical value in restoring the altered bowel ecology. Ginger also reduces inflammation in arthritis. **Grapefruit** contains pectin, the gelling agent present in the peel and membrane, which lowers cholesterol and facilitates blood flow in arteries. Pectin also appears to prevent blood clotting in arteries. **Squashes** have a long-established empirical role in improving digestive and absorptive functions. These vegetables are of special value in restoring bowel ecology and decreasing the bowel transit time (prevention of constipation and toxic effects of prolonged bowel transit time).

SELECTED MEDICINAL USES OF FOODS

Apple	Over-ripe apple poultice for bruises.
Beet Juice	Headache, dyspepsia
Celery/Potato Water	For stomach and bowel disorders, PMS, recurrent sore throat, and mood swings.
Cranberry juice	Urinary tract infections.
Cucumber/ Glycerine Lotion	Skin blemishes. Prepare with 3 ounces of juice and two teaspoons of glycerine.
Garlic	Hemorrhoids
Ginger	Chronic headache, chronic arthritis
Peach	Message skin of face with inside of peach for "peachy complexion".
Potato Water	Potato peel water for indigestion.
Parsley	For frequent urinary infection, Digestive problems
Raw Lemon juice	Two teaspoons raw juice before meals for respiratory and stomach maladies. Raw juice sprinkled on vegetables for indigestion.
Raw Potato	Apply to bruises and closed soft tissue injuries
Tomato Leaves Water	Joint, muscle and ligament problems.
Salt	Salt sauna for neuritis and muscle disorders

	Heat common salt, put it into cotton or flannel bag, place it over the painful areas.
Vinegar	Headache, fatigue, colds, anemia (Vinegar 1 tablespoon, honey 4 ounces, water 1 pint.

****

I close this chapter by reiterating criteria that separate life span from aging-oxidant foods.

* Life span foods are fresh and un-oxidized foods.
* Life span foods are free of toxic residues of chemical food processing.
* Life span foods are free of food incompatibilities.

We need to know all this. We also need to know about the skylights sprung over us by the marketing moguls of our food industry and by the nutrition professionals on their payroll.

Ethylene dibromide was used as fruit and vegetable fumigant. Sometime ago, many cases of serious toxicity caused by it were recognized. Government officials, under pressure from some consumer groups, banned the use of ethylene dibromide on fruit and vegetables. The chemistry wizards of fruit industry replaced ethylene dibromide with methyl bromide, even though they knew the latter is more volatile than the former. Methyl bromide outgases more, is more difficult to handle, and carries a greater risk of toxicity. That didn't seem to bother them. When people catch up with methyl bromide, they seemed to have reasoned, they will select another chemical. The cat-and-mouse game will continue. There will be more skylights.

Our national fast food outlets are now out to educate Americans about health. They tell us about the calories and salt and fat in their cheeseburgers, French fries, milk shakes and pies. What they do not tell us is far more important than what they do tell us. How much of the fat in the milk shake is oxidized, denatured fat? What kind of oils do they use to fry their French fries? What is the temperature of that oil? How long is that oil boiled before the French fries are dunked in it? These are the questions we need to ask them. These are the questions they are not prepared to answer. When I see vats of oil kept boiling for hours at end, I see whirlpools of toxic fats. When I see little children fed those French fries, I see orange-yellow streaks forming on the insides of their delicate arteries, and I see these streaks turning into plaques, heart attacks and stroke. This is not melodrama. I have seen too many of those streaks on the arteries of little children at autopsy. Do the money men of fast food industry know this? Do the nutrition experts on their payroll see the skylights of deception in the their "nutrition knowledge?" Do they care? Do the government officials know this? Do parents know this? The butterfly has no chance. *Or does it?*

Chapter 9

On Limbic Eating

We Are What We Observe

The ancients seemed to have intuitive insights into the relationships between food, health and disease. They recognized that the human frame was built of foods. It was fueled by foods. It was affected by foods. It responded to food. Indeed, it *was* food.

We Are What We Eat

The ancients exclaimed. They recognized that lungs exist to breathe in air to sustain life. They knew that the skin exists primarily to protect us from our environment though it absorbs many materials applied to it. Most importantly, they understood the role of the bowel in health and disease. They seemed to understand that the bowel is the primary interface between the body innards and the environment around it. All other body organs exist and function to facilitate conversion of food energy to other forms of energy necessary for life. Diseases are rooted in the bowel, they pronounced, in more than one way.

The ancients had much intuitive wisdom which we have turned our backs on. Rarely do we understand what we eat. Rarely do we attend to what happens to our food in the bowel. Rarely do we understand how the bowel responds to the food we put into it. Rarely do we recognize the relationship between what we eat and how we feel. When we fall ill, rarely do we attempt to link food with illness.

We Are What We Do Not Shit

Someone, afflicted with coprolalia, cried out, trying to translate the intuitive wisdom of the ancients into the contemporary vernacular.

We Are What We Absorb

We may say when we recognize the many threats to proper digestion and absorption of food material which we face today. Our bowel ecology is being threatened in many ways. With each meal, we get a bolus of pesticides, herbicides, preservatives and antibiotics. Toxic chemicals and heavy metals invade our biology every day. Our digestive enzymes are inactivated. Essential minerals, the life support of digestive enzymes, are often deficient. The local bowel immune system weakens. The gut becomes leaky and fails to keep out undigested foods, undesirable macromolecules and viruses, bacteria, yeast and parasites. The problems of digestion and absorption are interrelated and feed upon the other.

We Are What Our Plasma Membranes Are

We could say this to continue with this path of reasoning. After all, more important than absorption is how food molecules are used by plasma membranes (these membranes control all molecular events within the cells and in the cellular organelles, the tiniest structures within the cells).

We Are What Our Molecular Bioavailability Is

We may pursue this line of reasoning further. After all, molecules mean something only when they can function. Molecular function, in essence, is a matter of their availability in the metabolic molecular pathways.

But all this trivializes the intuitive wisdom of the ancients. Few things characterize our age more than complete dissociation between what we think we eat and what we believe the response of our bodies to our food is. The problem of our time is this: We have ceased to *observe*. What we lack is the capacity to observe the essential relatedness between our food and us, between what we eat and how we feel, between our patterns of eating and patterns of illness. The ancients did not have to confront as many assaults on their biology as we do today. If their external environment had been as devastated as ours, if their internal environment was as stressed and as polluted as ours, and if they had been as allergic to foods and as sensitive to chemicals as we are, they would most assuredly have exclaimed, "We are what we observe."

TWO BASIC OBSERVATIONS

The ancients made two basic observations about human

metabolism for which our nutrition and dieting experts, it seems to me, do not have much respect. I suspect this is so because these insights run counter to the profitability goals of our experts.

First,

the ancients knew that metabolism can be slowed down by fasting (the ancient equivalent of modern dieting). They knew and expounded the need for this during their periods of reflection, meditation, prayer and silence.

Second,

the ancients knew that metabolism can be accelerated by eating and with physical activity. Food fuels the furnace of human metabolism and exercise stokes its fire. Both truths are self-evident. All we have to do is to test them by *observing* the changes they produce.

Now consider what our dieting experts are advising us. They recommend dieting which down-regulates our catabolic enzymes (slows down the furnace). Or they recommend that we limit ourselves to their packaged foods. Or they advise us to ignore the diversity of foods in Nature and limit ourselves to one or two foods of their whims. Our dieting experts never ask us to observe the effects of their packaged diets on our total health for the whole life span.

Absence of Disease
Is Not Always Presence of Health

I wrote earlier that there is a critical difference between the states of an absence of disease and a presence of health. An increasing number of Americans know they are not healthy even when their physicians find the results of all the diagnostic tests performed to diagnose diseases to be negative. The biggest hurdle in the way of preventive medicine in the United States, it seems to me, is our failure to distinguish between the two states of the presence of disease and the absence of health. We physicians generally are very uncomfortable with early evolving disease. The state of "not healthy" caused by early molecular derangements in the body does not easily fit into our glib diagnostic labels. It is very convenient to deny the patient's suffering by labelling the problem all-in-the-head. This is an elegant expression for the physician to hide his ignorance of what really afflicts the patient.

In classical medical thinking, we dismiss a patient's suffering until the state of his ill health is advanced and our CAT and MRI scans and laboratories give us the *right* numbers and we diagnose a disease. The numbers determine what disease label we use for him and how hard we hit him with our drugs to "cure" him. I discuss in detail the intellectual handicaps of the practitioners of the prevailing drug medicine by disease-doctors in my book *The Cortical Monkey and Healing*.

A physician friend recently called me from Chicago and said,

> *"My wife has an abnormal protein spike in*
> *her blood. The hematologist at the medical*
> *school tells me there is nothing he can do*
> *now. Don't let a quack get his hands on her*
> *and give her vitamins, he told me. When it*
> *turns into myeloma (a type of bone cancer),*
> *we will hit her with chemotherapy."*

My friend had a choice of words for this hematologist which are not printable in a book like this. In the words of my friend Choua, nutritional medicine is a maligned discipline in medicine. There is a strange paradox here. Those who practice nutritional medicine find it most gratifying; those who do not find it worthless. Those who use herbs love it; those who do not hate it. This is a spurious debate. How can anyone find any therapy to be effective if he never uses it? How can anyone declare any therapy worthless if he has never tried it?

> *Taking supplements just gives you expensive*
> *urine. ..... But all the information is so*
> *contradictory. It's like trying to make your*
> *way through fog.*
> *Time* April 6, 1992

The first quote is from a physician well known for his disdain for nutritional medicine and his hatred of its practitioners. He, by his own admission, does not practice nutritional medicine. I suppose *Time* magazine ran his quote in their article because of his status as a head quack-buster, and not because his opinions are scientifically valid. Indeed, the

Time article included a compendium of studies documenting the value of nutrients in disease prevention and treatment. The second quote is of a non-scientist who intuitively knows toxic pollutants that surround us *must* be dangerous to our biology, and that the body cannot be healed with synthetic drugs. Injured tissues must rely on nutrients for healing. Here is the crux of the problem: Physicians who should know better (they are supposed to study the impact of nutrients and toxins on human biology) look down on nutritional medicine; lay people who do not know the science of the structure and function of nutrient molecules yearn for nutritional approaches to good health and absence of disease.

Young Butterflies Learn

Martha Weiss of University of Arizona studied how the changing colors of *Lantana* flowers influence feeding patterns of butterflies. The flowers open yellow, turn orange the next day and then red for the remaing seven days. Weiss observed that older butterflies prefer yellow flowers that are rich in necter and ready to pollinate. The young butterflies, by contrast, first visit red and yellow flowers equally and then learn to favor yellow flowers.

The plant esssentially 'teaches' the insect to focus its attention on sexually active and rewarding flowers," she says.

Science News 142:186; 1992

The young butterflies learn, so do children. Flowers teach the young butterflies. Who teaches little children?

Information or Disinformation

There are two important problems in nutrition education in the United States today.

First,

two brands of nutrition knowledge exist today. There is a brand of nutrition knowledge promulgated by those who practice nutritional medicine and who prevent and treat diseases with nutrients. The other is a brand of nutrition science put forth by physicians who are up on their statistics for diseases and drugs, and are down on nutritional medicine which they consider as quackery. They have sharp tongues, weild great power at medical boards, and far outnumber nutritionist-physicians. The American people are uncertain as to whose word they should accept, the highly visible majority of mainstream docs or a weak small minority of holistic docs.

Second,

the nutritionist-physicians in the first group are actively harassed by our medical boards. The drug-doctors in the second category are strongly backed by the enormous financial muscle of our drug and food industries. The result is that the voice and experience of knowledgeable nutritionist-physicians are lost. The thunderous voices of the food and drug industries and ignorance of the general medical profession become partners in the crimes perpetrated against the nutrition and health of Americans.

On last Eid (a Muslim religious holiday), I had lunch at

my sister Quanita's home. There were several other physicians present. Three physician friends of my age had recently undergone coronary angioplasty for advanced heart disease. Understandably, other physicians in the same age group were very concerned about what was happening to our peers. I saw one of them pick food from the table under close scrutiny of his wife who is also a physician. My friend took meager portions of food, avoiding what his wife thought were "fatty" foods. Neither of them has any concept of good natural fats and toxic denatured fats. To them, fats are fats. They subscribe to the party line. Cholesterol is bad. Why? Because the high priests of American medicine who consider nutritional medicine quackery say so. I reflected on their plight as I watched the husband and wife continue their silent struggle. How many adrenaline and other aging-oxidant molecules do they produce in their bodies by their struggle at each meal time? How often do they constrict their coronary arteries worrying about cholesterol?

Most of the time when I do an autopsy on people who die within six to eight hours of their heart attacks, I do not find blood clots in their arteries. So how did these people die? By constricting and closing off their coronary arteries. I wondered if my physician friends knew this. I wondered if they knew anything about down-regulated, clogged enzymatic pathways that cause heart attacks. I wondered if they were aware that enzymes can be up-regulated with limbic listening and with limbic exercise. What an irony! To avoid the innocent molecule of cholesterol, they produce a surge of the aging-oxidant molecules of denial, anger and stress.

How can we physicians advise our patients correctly if we ourselves are ignorant of what is and what is not important in nutrition. All fats are not the villain in the heart story. Toxic fats are. How much food we eat is not important. What kind of foods we eat is important. Is the food laced with aging-oxidant molecules? Is it largely composed of life span foods? Are our enzymes clogged? Are our enzymes up-regulated? What can we do to up-regulate our clogged enzymes? These are the critical questions. The American College of Cardiology and the cardiac surgery community do not much care for such notions of metabolism, health and disease. Our cardiac surgeons hate chelation therapy. It takes their scalpel business away from them. They approach heart disease as a plumbing problem.

Looking at heart disease as a plumbing problem, I must concede, is very enriching for our cardiologists and cardiac surgeons. What does it do for the people struck with heart disease? We physicians are too busy doling out our wonder drugs to worry about such questions. Our drug therapies do serve one purpose though: They assure us that people with heart disease have no real chance of reversing their disease.

In the chapter, Life Span Food Choices, I give criteria for separating information from misinformation. I reiterate here four essential criteria for making this distinction:

First,

sound scientific information about nutrients must be based upon the basic knowledge of the structure and function of molecules. This may seem difficult for the person without a science background, but it need not be. I discuss the basic concept of life span molecules and aging-oxidant molecules in this book in a way that, I believe, can serve as a good primer for the non-scientist.

Second,

we need to know where the nutritional advice is coming from. Is nutritional advice coming from people who practice nutritional medicine? Do they treat diseases with nutrients? Do they practice preventive medicine? Example: Would I take my nutrition information from the airline advertisements of a famous heart surgery center in Texas? I know for a fact that no physician at that center practices nutritional medicine. No one at that center practices preventive medicine. How did they build their huge medical center? By operating on people or by teaching them how to get well and stay well without surgery? Similarly, "nutrition science" promoted by fast food merchants and the experts of the food industry (doctors on their payroll) is more often than made up of self-serving and misleading half-truths.

Third.

the popular mice and medical student "research" studies, with rare exceptions, are worthless. We are not interested in what oat bran fed to 19 medical students for four weeks does to their blood cholesterol levels, especially when such research studies do not tell us how much this bran interferes in the absorption of minerals essential for the health of the heart. We are interested in the science of the basic structure and function of molecules. We are interested in holistic molecular relatedness in human biology. And we are interested in the optimal health of a person for his entire life span.

Fourth,

and most emphatically, we must categorically reject the science of those nutrition experts who, by their own admission, do not practice nutritional medicine and who are very vocal in denouncing those who do. Vitamin therapy is a way of making expensive urine, they cry out. I do not begrudge them their "science" of the naming diseases and suppressing symptoms with drugs, but clearly I reject their claims to expertise in an area in which, again by their own admission, they have no true-to-life experience.

Faced with the pervasive contradictions in available nutrition knowledge, the general reader has *no choice but to learn the basics of life chemistry so he can see through the nutrition science of the practitioners of drug medicine and their bias against nutrients.* Drugs, I reiterate, are aging-oxidant molecules, though they serve as lifesaving molecules in acute diseases. In chronic diseases, drugs are poor substitutes for therapies based on life span molecules.

It seems to me that if we make these basic considerations the foundation of our knowledge of practical nutrition, it is not very difficult for anyone to have a workable philosophy of nutrition for the entire life span. People without a science background are generally intimidated by the scientific jargon. In the chapter, Life Span Food Choices, I give the basics of the essential chemistry of life in a simplified manner. I repeat my comments about the basic equation of life and my theory of spontaneity of oxidation as the true nature of the aging process in man several times for the general reader because this is my essential message.

Food Incompatibility
and Abnormal Bowel Responses

No discussion of the relationship of food to the human condition can be complete without some comments about food incompatibility and abnormal bowel responses to food. I make some essential points about this subject before outlining some steps for limbic eating.

When the nose weeps, allergy is evident to everyone. When the bowel cries out with cramps, we do not think of bowel allergy or food reactions. We try to simply smother the bowel with drugs. When the eyes burn, we look for toxic pollutants in the air. When the heart hurts (and palpitates), we do not think of chemical sensitivity but try to simply suppress the symptoms with drugs.

The single most important cause of fatigue in my experience is food and mold allergy. Every one of my patients with chronic fatigue syndrome has food incompatibilities. Problems of mood, memory and mentation can often be relieved by proper management of food incompatibilities. I have never seen a patient with chronic colitis who could not be proven to have food allergy with appropriate food allergy tests. Most patients with asthma and the vast majority of young patients with arthritis have food allergy. I do not recall ever seeing a patient with autoimmune disease who was not food or mold allergic. All practitioners of environmental medicine and physician-nutritionists will readily agree to all this. Regrettably, there are physicians who dismiss the problem of food incompatibility and allergy as problems in the head. Indeed, some textbooks of pediatrics still consider the incidence of food allergy among children as quite low.

There is another paradox here. Food incompatibilities and abnormal bowel responses to food are simple problems for some professionals and exceedingly complex for others. Those who look for allergy find it and know that it is an extremely common problem. Those who do not, tend to think food allergy is very rare. They continue to treat with drugs many cases of food incompatibility that they regard as diseases of idiopathic origin. The term idiopathic is an elegant expression. It means we do not know its cause. The problem here is that after we call something idiopathic, we stop looking for the real cause. The term idiopathic does not tell anything to us physicians and it hides much from our patients.

SIX ESSENTIALS OF FOOD INCOMPATIBILITY

The presence of food incompatibilities cannot be understood without understanding six essential facets of these problems.

First,

an individual's genetic make-up programs him to react to his environment to a lesser or greater degree. Both the fixed and cyclical types of food allergy described below tend to run in families. Indeed, if both parents have allergic genes, the children have about a 90% chance of being allergic as well.

Second,

the degree to which a person is exposed to a given food affects the degree of food incompatibility. Even when an individual has allergic genes, we would not expect him to show reactions if he is not exposed to that food. Indeed, this happens. The primary reason why allergic children are more often than not allergic to dairy products is that they are fed dairy products every day, sometimes several times during the same day. The same holds for wheat, corn and egg. Milk-allergic infants who are put on soy formulas exclusively often develop partial tolerance to milk but become sensitive to soy. In other words, we switch our sensitivities as we switch our foods. That is why rotation in diet is the *centerpiece* of a proper management plan for food incompatibilities.

Generally, people do not show many incompatibilities to vegetables. There are, however, some exceptions. Sometime ago I saw a very high electrodermal response to broccoli in a woman. That came as a surprise to me. I found out she had eaten broccoli three times a day for the last eight years. The reason: She had a colon cancer removed eight years previously and was advised to eat broccoli every day. She did so religiously. What was the positive electrodermal test to broccoli telling her? That even a good anticancer food like broccoli must not be eaten every day.

Third,

the total burden an individual carries on his biology has

great impact on his state of health. I have seen patients who can eat and tolerate beef well in a restaurant by the sea after a day of leisure on a beach. Yet they react badly to beef when they eat it in a city restaurant after a stressful day at work. People often develop new incompatibilities after viral infections and exposure to chemicals. This is sometimes called a *spreading phenomenon*. The reasons for this are self-evident: Allergic people have more reactions when they are under multiple biologic stresses. The reverse of this also pertains. When patients with chronic immune disorders get better, they often lose many of their food incompatibilities.

Fourth,

the "biologic carrying capacity" of an individual determines the degree to which biologic stressors cause adverse health effects. I commonly see otherwise healthy people who show very high levels of allergy-causing IgE antibodies and yet they suffer only minor allergy symptoms, while others, who suffer from chronic health disorders, have very low levels of such antibodies but develop severe allergic symptoms. The concept of total biologic burden on an individual is being increasingly recognized; the issue of the carrying capacity of the person, by contrast, is rarely understood.

Fifth,

the realization of the full impact of an individual's food incompatibilities only comes *after* he has cleared his system of incompatible foods. This is a point of enormous practical importance. Almost every day I see people who became aware of their food incompatibilities only after they had eliminated incompatible foods for several weeks. It is difficult, if not impossible, to relate incompatibility reactions to foods that cause them if a person suffers from those reactions all the time. A test period of elimination of incompatible foods must precede the food challenge — a body must be cleansed of incriminated foods before the cause-and effect can be clearly discerned. As an analogy, it is hard to appreciate classical music if one stands on top of a subway vent when the trains are rushing by below him. He has to let the train pass by before he can hear the music.

Nothing encourages me more than a child's telling me of his discovery that some foods make him feel bad. In general, children with food incompatibilities initially fight hard to resist any changes in their food. They crave the very foods to which they react. After some weeks or months, they begin to feel better, and then comes Thanksgiving. They eat sugar and incompatible foods and react. Some days later, they begin to clear and feel better, and the Christmas arrives. They nosedive again. This cycle of feeling good on healthy foods and feeling sick with incompatible foods repeats itself a few times before a six-year-old child learns what many physicians often do not: Incompatible foods make people unwell.

How many times have I seen people with an impossible sweet tooth who reach a state of total intolerance to desserts? How often have I seen people with impossible dependence on caffeine completely give up coffee? How often have I seen children who practically lived on orange juice become averse to it? These are common observations for me and my colleagues in nutritional medicine.

Sixth,

there is a phenomenon of paradoxical food reactions. JK, an engineer in early forties, consulted me for chronic fatigue, muscle weakness, severe abdominal bloating and cramps, mood swings, mental confusion and short-term memory loss, and depression. He knew he was sensitive to dairy, sugar and many other foods. He also had mold and chemical sensitivities. As happens frequently in patients who suffer from this fell disorder, he felt rapid improvement initially with treatment and then suffered a relapse. One day, he said,

"Dr. Ali, I don't understand this. During the last three days, I have been experimenting with foods as you suggested. You know I actually felt better after I ate ice cream, and felt drained of energy after I drank fresh vegetable juice."

This is an excellent case study of what I call paradoxical food reactions. Such reactions are seen during early stages of management of food incompatibility and allergy, and represent abnormal body responses that are at variance with those expected under normal expectations. Paradoxical food responses are reflections of varying patterns of adaptation, nonadaptation, maladaptation, de-adaptations and, finally, nonadapated state of exhaustion.

Adaptation, and the abnormalities of adaptation, are the

processes by which an organisms strives to preserve its health in the face of an acute or chronic challenge (physiological, biochemical or emotional stressors). Nonadaptation is the initial state of alarm — the commonly recognized state of stress reaction. Adaptation is the state of masked responses — the stressor causes the change, but the change remains hidden as the body calls up its reserves. Maladaptation is a state of ill-health caused when the stressor overwhelms the adaptive capability of the organism. The final state is that of exhaustion — the organism no longer can respond to the stressors, and a state of collapse follows.

Food incompatibility reactions are usually excitatory initially, but can pass into inhibitory responses as the problem becomes deeper. This phenomenon is observed in a reverse order during recovery. I believe this phenomenon was the primary basis of the observation made by the ancients that on the way out of a chronic illness, a patient often suffers from the problems he faced on his way into the disease. Physicians who practice nutritional medicine know such responses well. They also know that these reactions do not occur after successful management of food incompatibilities.

Cortical Habits, Limbic Habits

Is eating well always a struggle? How long do we need to closely follow our food plans? Are we condemned to keep food diaries for ever? Remember what we ate yesterday so we can rotate our foods today? Will we always offend our senses by reading food labels? Will denial be the way of life? Punishment at each meal time?

Eat what is best for you;
habit will make it agreeable.

Children with hyperactivity syndrome and attention deficit disorders caused by food incompatibilities give eloquent answer to these questions. They paraphrase Aristotle's words in their down-to-earth answers to my questions during my follow-up visits with them. Food craving is the flip-side of the coin of food incompatibility. Preaching a child with sugar addiction to stay from sugar, in many ways, is akin to asking a cocaine addict to say 'No' to his daily fix. Still, I see this every day. Sometimes it takes weeks, sometimes months, but it does happen. With proper professional support and gentle and persistent parental guidance, children do learn the relationship between their food and their condition. They learn to *know* the signals from their tissues, cells and molecules. With time, eating what they like to eat becomes the same thing as eating what they need to eat. This is limbic eating. There is no more any need to keep food diaries, hassle of choosing alternative foods, fretting about rotation. All this is done effortlessly and naturally, at some higher visceral-intuitive level. The cortical monkey relinquishes its hold. Limbic habits replace cortical habits.

Decisions! Decisions! Decisions!

Some new patients arrive for consultation with me armed heavily with notions of food families, cross-reactivities among foods, food elimination and rotation, yeast-free diets and no-sugar diets. I do not know how much stress they were under before they put themselves on special diets, but I readily recognize the stress caused by restrictive diets. It often reminds me of a story my brother used to tell.

A man was about to retire after thirty years of service in a fruit-packing plant. His job required him to pick damaged apples from a conveyer belt before they were packed into boxes. Some years before he was to retire, he started calling his day of retirement a day of deliverance. As his retirement day neared, his talk about his deliverance day became incessant and annoying. His family and friends bore all that with good grace. The day before retirement, his excitement peaked and his words became unbearable for everyone around him. A friend got very irritated and said, "I know this is a big day for you. But you should really calm down."

"But you don't understand," He beamed.

"I understand," the friend responded, "you have been looking forward to this day for a long time. "

"No! No! You don't understand," he answered excitedly.

"Calm down. Such excitement is not healthy," the friend admonished.

"No! No! You don't understand."

"Understand what? What is there to understand anyway?

You are retiring and you will a lot of free time" The friend replied with irritation.

"It's not about leisure time. You don't understand at all," the man grinned broadly.

"If it is not leisure, what else is it? You will not have to go to work."

"No!"

"You will travel?"

"No!"

"So then what is it? All you did was pick damaged apples from the conveyer belt."

"That's it! It is about decisions!"

"Decisions?" The friend was incredulous.

"Yes! Decisions! Decisions! Decisions!"

****

Pursuit of perfection can be paralyzing. It is truer in matters of nutrition and health — it seems to me — than in any other area. What is required is an intuitive-visceral sense of what should be eaten and what may be declined among foods. Such a sense follows a true understanding of the sound scientific knowledge of nutrients, naturally and effortlessly. Once we know something about the effects of our foods on our condition, we cannot not know it.

Fixed and Cyclical Food Allergy

Food allergy is a misunderstood subject. The principal reason for this is the failure of many people to understand the difference between two distinct types of food allergy and reactions: fixed food allergy and cyclical food allergy.

Fixed food allergy is the type of allergy in which each exposure to the allergic food causes an allergic reaction. Examples: milk asthma, peanut hives, swelling of lips after eating oranges, headache after eating corn and other such reactions. The individual knows that he will react each time he eats the offending food. The diagnosis of this type of allergy is established by the individual's own experience. It does not require allergy tests, except as a confirmatory test.

Cyclical food allergy is an altogether different type of allergy reaction. It often goes unrecognized, both by the individual and his physician. Sometimes the person observes a certain reaction, suspects he might be reacting to something in his food but is unable to pinpoint the offending food. Examples: A person feels tired after eating wheat: a person gets a headache the morning after eating a chocolate cake at dinner or experiences mood swings several hours after ingesting a particular food.

Cyclical food reactions may occur within five days after eating the food. Not uncommonly, the allergic reaction is evoked by a breakdown product of the food. There are people who tolerate raw milk but not pasteurized milk and there are those who cannot drink raw milk but experience no difficulty with pasteurized milk. Twice I personally developed a serious allergy reaction to carrot juice with widespread hives, swelling around my eyes and heart palpitations (which I successfully controlled within several minutes with autoregulation). Yet I can eat cooked carrots without any reactions.

A reliable way of diagnosing food allergy and abnormal bowel responses to foods is by the method of elimination and provocation. In this method, a food suspecting of causing allergy is eliminated from the diet for a minimum of five days, and is then eaten as a challenge. The individual then specifically looks for the development of symptoms that he has experienced in the past. A pulse count before and after the food test may be helpful. Similarly, peak flow measurements for persons with asthma or wheezing are good indications of the presence of an allergic reaction. However, elimination-provocation method is time-consuming and not very useful for most clinical situations.

Laboratory Tests for Food Incompatibility

There is no single perfect test for food allergy and abnormal bowel responses to food. In my own medical practice, I use a combination of micro-elisa assay for IgE antibodies and electrodermal conductance tests. Less commonly, I do provocation/neutralization tests for diagnosis.

My research colleague, Madhava Ramanarayanan, Ph.D., and I first introduced the micro-elisa assay for food, mold and pollen allergy in 1979 and 1980. During the next few years, we published extensive data about its clinical usefulness in a series of papers (some selected citations follow this section). During my work as a hospital pathologist over the last 25 years, I have had the opportunity to examine over 12,000 biopsies of the bowel and stomach for noncancerous diseases. In my clinical practice I have seen a very large number of patients with allergy, immune and degenerative diseases, and chronic bowel disorders. The following paragraphs describe my preference for diagnostic tests for food allergy and abnormal bowel responses to ingested food.

Micro-elisa assay for IgE antibodies with specificity for food, mold and pollen allergens is, in my judgment, the best starting point. It is essential that such testing be done by experienced and knowledgeable laboratory staff. Diagnostic intracutaneous skin tests and provocation/neutralization appear to be equally good in experienced hands.

Another commonly used blood test for allergy diagnosis is the assay for measurement of IgG antibodies with specificity for food allergens. Soon after we developed the first micro-elisa assay for IgE antibodies, my colleague Dr. Ramanarayanan and I developed a micro-elisa assay for IgG antibodies. After extensive laboratory and clinical evaluation, we concluded that the IgG assay is not a suitable test for allergy diagnosis. This assay, however, is an excellent test for assessing the immune response of the patient to allergy desensitization treatment. I routinely use IgG test for this purpose. IgG antibodies, with extremely rare exceptions, are protective antibodies. These antibodies function as "good" antibodies (G for good) and block the "evil", allergy-causing IgE antibodies (E for evil).

Tests for blood levels of histamine do not give information about specific food allergies. Circulating immune complexes with specificity for incriminated foods can be used with good results, but these are research tests and are generally not available for clinical work. Some kinesiologists report good results with diagnosis of food allergy made with their techniques. In my own clinical work, a few patients previously treated by others with methods of kinesiology report good results. Most patients, however, do not report satisfactory results. I am unable to comment on this method any further.

The electrodermal conductance technology for detection of food incompatibilities is of great value in the clinical practice of nutritional medicine. I do not know of a *perfect* technology in medicine, and this technology is no exception. It is easy for an inexperienced individual to make mistakes with his use of electrodes and the acupuncture sensitivity point. However, the results in experienced hands are most impressive. Although our understanding of the electromagnetic principles underlying this technology is limited, I have been very impressed with the clinical results observed with information obtained with this detection approach. It separates with a fairly high degree of accuracy the foods that "agree" with us in a biochemical and an electromagnetic sense and those that do not. Such information is extremely valuable in nutritional planning for individual patients.

In one of my studies, I observed a very high correlation between food incompatibility diagnosed with an IgE micro-Elisa assay for antibodies in blood and that detected with electrodermal conductance. The latter test was positive in almost all cases when the blood test was positive, and further detected incompatibilities in many cases in which the blood test turned out to be negative (Am J Clin Pathol 91:357; 1989).

References for Allergy Tests

Ali, M. Otolaryng Head Neck Surg. 87:45; 1979.
Ali, M. et al Clinical Allergy 10:203; 1980.
Ali, M. Ramanarayanan et al Am J Clin Path 81:591; 1984.
Ali, M. Ramanarayanan et al Am J Clin Path 80:290; 1983.
Ali, M. Ramanarayanan et al Annals of Allergy 45:63; 1980
Ali, M. Clinical Ecology 3:68; 1986.
Ali, M. Am J Clin Pathol 91:357; 1989

Ways to Limbic Eating

I am not a martyr. I do not believe in martyrdom at mealtime. When people honor me by asking me to be their physician, I do not recommend that they become martyrs either.

I know what it means to be limbic in eating. To be limbic is to be free. Free from the need to do the *right* things. Free of plans. Free of censor. Free of the need to know. In limbic eating, a person does not eat well to stay healthy or slim. He eats to sustain himself, naturally and effortlessly, and without martyrdom. The food choices come from within. It may seem improbable to some, but it is possible to eat limbically even at airports.

This book is about the "language of silence," about limbic openness, and about *knowing* something about the human condition. I return to these subjects frequently for emphasis. I recognize this repetition may be disagreeable to some readers, but I also recognize limbic eating cannot be *received* without these elements.

Extensive clinical work has convinced me that we cannot eat limbically by counting calories, eating whole bread and using margarine to lower saturated fats. There is more, much more, to eating for the life span than following the "sound bite" advice on nutrition. What makes for good TV does not make for good eating for the life span.

Following, I give a summary of steps that can, with time,

free us from cortical clutter of foods lead us to limbic eating with visceral-intuitive wisdom of our enzymes and nutrients.

FIRST, WE MUST HAVE A SENSE OF WHAT IS REAL IN NUTRITION AND WHAT IS NOT

The medical literature about nutrition at its face value is so conflicting and contradictory that it is very close to being worthless. So the first order of business in nutrition must be to separate information from disinformation. I give my criteria for making this distinction earlier in this chapter.

Nutrition is a good word. Dieting is a bad word. We are interested in nutritional philosophy. We are not interested in nutritional cultism. Dieting is a strategy of denial. The flip side of this coin, I wrote earlier in the book, is euphoria of eating. It is far easier to bring new foods in rather than struggle with taking foods out of our nutritional plan. Food cultism is a misdirected struggle to dissolve misunderstood anguish.

Being a Skunk in Someone's Garden Party

When some one is gracious enough to offer us his company and a special meal, it is not the time to preach to him about the virtues of good foods and the evils of bad foods. It is a time for joy. A time for sharing. A time for gratitude. A time for *being*. Special foods on special occasions are foods for the moment. If our enzymes are optimally up-regulated, an occasional food *indulgence* is of no concern. If our enzymes are down-regulated, even a sparse meal clogs the molecular wheels of our metabolism. If we eat well most of the time, our enzymes can handle an occasional workout. There is no defense for being a skunk in someone's garden party. Fixed food allergy for me is the only acceptable reason for refusing special foods on special occasions.

The value of proper professional guidance is paramount. Nutrient supplements are absolutely *essential* to counterbalance the avalanche of aging-oxidant molecules in our internal and external environments. Those who say nutrients prescribed by knowledgeable physicians only give expensive urine are sadly misinformed. Nutrition books like this are valuable for providing reliable knowledge. However, no book can be a true substitute for a knowledgeable and caring professional. In the Appendix, I include addresses of the American Academy of Environmental Medicine, the American College of Advancement in Medicine, the Foundation for Innovations in Medicine and various other physician associations dedicated to preventive medicine. Members of these organizations are generally familiar with the principles and practice of nutritional medicine as outlined in this volume.

SECOND, WE MUST KNOW WHAT A GOOD MEAL IS

What is a good meal? Is this a simple question? It is also

one of the most profound questions in the entire field of nutrition. Here is my definition of a good meal:

- A good meal is a meal that leaves us light and energetic after we finish it.
- A good meal is a meal that sustains us with vigor and vitality till   the next meal.
- A good meal, as the ancients proclaimed, is a meal that stops just short of full satiety and does not cause undue fullness in the stomach.
- A good meal is a meal that does not plunge us into molecular roller-coasters (rapid disabling hypoglycemic-hyperglycemic shifts, adrenaline surges, and acetylcholine and other neurotransmitter flashes).
- A good meal is a meal that supports our biology with life span molecules.
- A good meal is a meal that does not violate our biology with aging-oxidant molecules.
- A good meal is a meal that contains uninjured foods.
- A good meal is a meal that protects us against molecular injury to our molecules, cells and organs.
- A good meal is a meal that we can *respect.*
- A good meal is a meal that *respects* us.

Life Span Meals

Some meals sustain the human life span. I call these "life

span meals." Some other meals threaten the human life span. I call these meals "aging-oxidant meals." I give my criteria for dividing foods into these two categories in the chapter, Life Span Food Choices. Here I reiterate briefly the main criteria for differentiating these meals.

To be considered a life span meals, a meal must support life span molecules and counter aging-oxidant molecules. They should support the reductive (antioxidant) arm of the basic redox reaction in human biology. They should be predominantly alkaline ash foods, and should reduce the acidity or neutralize acidotic stress on human metabolism. They should yield their energy in a time-release fashion and prevent sudden molecular highs and molecular lows. They should prevent molecular roller coasters (sudden highs and lows of rapid hypoglycemic-hyperglycemic shifts, sudden adrenaline surges, cholinergic crises and other related molecular events).

AGING-OXIDANT MEALS

The primary metabolic effects of these meals are oxidant in nature. These meals cause or promote oxidation of other foods. They cause or increase acidotic stress on human metabolism. They release their energy in sudden bursts, and they cause or promote molecular roller coasters.

Let us consider an example of an "aging-oxidant meal". This meal includes a top-of-the-line hamburger, French fries and cookies from one of the leading national hamburger outlets.

The following table dramatically shows the enormous biologic burden of this meal on a teenager.

	Calories	Fat	Sodium
Hamburger	510	252 Cal	1110 mg
French Fries	400	188 Cal	200 mg
Cookies	330	135 Cal	289 mg
TOTAL	1240	675 Cal	1599 mg

This meal is in reality a toxic meal, an antimeal. It damages the enzymatic pathways of the innocent, unsuspecting teenager in many ways.

First,

it puts a massive load of calories on his metabolism.

Second,

it is laced with toxic fats that clog his molecular pathways of fat metabolism.

Third,

it puts an enormous burden of salt on his cellular metabolism and kidneys.

Fourth,

it throws him into hyperglycemic-hypoglycemic roller coasters, with associated rapid insulin and adrenaline surges.

Fifth,

it puts him in double jeopardy of vitamin and mineral depletion. This meal almost completely robs him of all vitamins and minerals, such as magnesium, potassium, sulfur, calcium, zinc and molybdenum. Further, the toxic calories in this meal force the body to use up its meager reserves of such vital nutrients.

The teenager may recognize that such a meal makes him sluggish, but he is not likely to understand the long-term dire consequences of such metabolic insults.

Sugar and salt such in massive quantities are poisons for the heart, arteries, kidneys and brain. And the tragedy of "nutritional value" of this meal does not end there. The real tragedy is that this meal is laced with toxic fats. French fries are prepared by dunking them in a boiling cesspool of toxic cyclic peroxides of fats and trans fatty acids. Salt is a much bigger cause of sugar craving than is realized by most people. Some decades later, our teenager will have clogged arteries, a heart weakened with suffocation, sluggish legs (and amputation if he is not lucky), kidney failure and limbs paralyzed with strokes. Then our Star Wars medicine will offer him its high-tech tools. Our cardiologists will prescribe a slew of drugs (which will assure that his clogged arteries remain clogged), and our cardiac surgeons will want to bypass his clogged arteries. Both groups will forcefully warn him against quacks who practice nutritional medicine and offer nutrient therapies and chelation. The promise of Star Wars medicine will have been delivered.

A LIFE SPAN MEAL

Now let us consider an example of a life span meal. It includes chicken curry, brown rice, steamed (or stir-fried) vegetables and a peach (or fresh fruit pieces put in apple juice thickened with kuzu). The following table shows the nutritional profile of this meal.

	Calories	Fats	Salt
Chicken	153	36	51 Mg
Brown Rice	178	9	0 Mg
Vegetables	131	0.2	33 Mg
Fruit	37	0	0 Mg
TOTAL	399	45	84 Mg

The above table tells only part of the story. This life span meal is very rich in minerals, vitamins, life span calories and is almost devoid of any toxic fats.

I have carefully considered the issues of toxic fats, salt and fat overload and nutrient density in dividing foods into the four groups given in the chapter, Life Span Food Choices. It is tragic how often so many professionals mindlessly talk about the caloric value of food without any regard to how many of its calories are life span calories and how many are aging-oxidant calories. I include below the caloric value of foods only as a matter of general information. I reiterate here what I wrote earlier in this volume: Life span nutrition is not about counting calories. It is a philosophy of nutrition. It is the study of the relationship between food and the human condition. A teaspoon of sugar contains 4 grams of sugar, and a tablespoon 16 grams. The following table of the caloric value of foods is included here for general information of the reader.

Carbohydrates	4.0	Calories per gram
Proteins	4.1	Calories per gram
Fats	9.0	Calories per gram

THIRD, WE GO SLOWLY AND STEADILY

Sudden changes in eating habits rarely give good results. Sudden changes are cortical devices. Slow and sustained changes are limbic responses.

* We need not be martyrs every time we eat.
* We need not abuse our gut each time we eat.

* We need not get a high while we eat.
* We need not get a low after we eat.

We Go Naturally

We need to:

Know our life span foods and aging-oxidant foods.

Know our food allergies and abnormal bowel responses.

Know what metabolic roller coasters are, how they are caused, how they stress our metabolism, and how we can avoid them.

Avoid foods that keep; what bugs won't eat cannot be much good for us.

Eat foods that spoil before they spoil. Foods have their own life spans. Foods spoil when high-energy molecules disintegrate.

Recognize our major antinutrients that pass as nutrients: white sugar, white flour, white rice, and white oils.

Take judicious and balanced nutrient supplements with regularity.

Read labels. (Though this becomes unnecessary as we recognize life span foods at an intuitive-visceral level.

Over the years, manufacturers have managed to manipulate virtually every listing on packaged foods — serving size, fat and sodium contents, and even chemical additives — so as to conceal rather than reveal nutritional land mines.

Harvard Health Letter May 1992.

How bad can the labeling be? The answer: really bad. For example, a turkey frankfurter labeled "80% fat free" actually carries 76% of its calories in fats. As shown in the preceding table, one gram of fat contains more than twice as many calories as one gram of protein and carbohydrates (9 versus 4.1 and 4 per gram).

Reading labels, however, is not for the limbic eater. It is necessary only in the beginning as a person begins to develop a philosophy of nutrition. After a while the limbic sense takes over. There is no yearning for aging-oxidant foods. As for the nutrient supplements, I include some general recommendations for basic nutrient supplementation at the end of this chapter. I repeat, there is no substitute for the advice of a caring physician who is well-versed in the principles and practice of nutritional medicine. And there is no point in seeking advice on this subject from physicians who do not practice nutritional medicine.

Chemicals Are Cellular Diuretics

Chemicals dry out the cells.

Cellular aging causes several well-defined changes in the cell. The water content of the cell diminishes, and the fat content increases. Environmental toxins poke holes in the cell membrane. The cell wall is literally shot-full-of-holes. I indicate in the chapter Life Span Food Choices how magnesium and potassium hemorrhage out and calcium floods the cell innards when the cell membrane is damaged. Deficiency of magnesium and potassium in the cells slows down the cellular enzymes. Extra calcium within the cells further poisons these enzymes. The molecular pathways within the cells are clogged. The cell suffocates. This is the true nature of what I call accelerated aging.

FOURTH, WE DISCOVER THE FREQUENCY OF EATING THAT IS RIGHT FOR US

Frequency of meals is an important issue for many people. Hypoglycemia (low blood sugar levels) is a pervasive but very misunderstood health disorder in America today.

Life in America is characterized by accelerated molecular oxidative stress on human biology. My patients have given me an important insight into the metabolic consequences of this phenomenon. *Three body organs bear the brunt of accelerated oxidative molecular damage: the thyroid gland, the pancreas and the adrenal gland.* This, in my judgment, is the real reason why the disorders of underactive thyroid (hypothyroidism), low blood sugar (hypoglycemia) and *functional* derangements of the adrenal gland (the chronic stress syndrome) are so pervasive in America. Sad to say, these problems are also rapidly becoming pervasive in other parts of planet Earth. Environmental pollutants carry no prejudice.

Hypoglycemia Is A Misunderstood Phenomenon

Hypoglycemia is a widely misunderstood and mismanaged health disorder. I discuss this subject later in this chapter. The essential element as it pertains to our discussion of the frequency and size of our meals is the avoidance of molecular roller coasters caused by rapid highs and lows in blood levels of sugar, adrenaline and other stress molecules, and acetylcholine and other neurotransmitter molecules. *We must never miss breakfast.* Missing breakfast and having a doughnut and coffee at mid-morning is asking for trouble. I cannot overstate the case for regular meals at regular times. Many people with hypoglycemia need five or six small meals rather three large ones to avoid molecular roller coasters.

FIFTH, WE MUST KNOW OUR FOOD INCOMPATIBILITIES AND ABNORMAL BOWEL RESPONSES

The prevailing notions of food incompatibility and allergy

among the practitioners of drug medicine are pathetically in error. Except for physicians who practice nutritional medicine, the concept of food incompatibility simply does not exist among the physcian community. Allergy is narrowly defined as reactions caused by foods only when specific antibodies are present; its presence is only accepted when it can be proven with a positive skin test or by IgE antibody tests. This limited view of the relationship between foods and ill health is hardly of any value to people concerned about their health.

We must know our food incompatibilities and our abnormal bowel responses to food. The case for proper diagnosis and management of food allergy and abnormal bowel responses cannot be overstated. This is essential for people with allergy. This is also advisable for people who do not suffer from classical allergy symptoms. I discussed this subject earlier in this chapter.

Once We Know,
We Cannot Not Know

This is the essence of food allergy and abnormal bowel responses. How often do I see patients with milk asthma who are on multiple drugs for breathing and whose food allergy remains undiagnosed? How often do I see little children who become hyperactive after they eat sugary snacks and who are given drugs for discipline? How often do I see patients whose "tension" headache is caused by mold allergy but is suppressed with painkillers, only to return with greater intensity? How often do I see patients who react to formaldehyde and are told it is "all in their heads?"

Milk allergic persons should remember that *cow's milk is good for baby cows and goat's milk for baby goats.* Man is the only animal who drinks milk all his life, and not from his own mother. Pet animals drink milk to keep their masters happy. Dairy products are good for the dairy industry but not always for people. The so-called calcium argument is a spurious issue. There are many other excellent sources of calcium. Milk is by far the most prevalent food allergen.

SIXTH, WE MUST UNDERSTAND MOLECULAR UNIQUENESS AND RELATEDNESS

We are all unique individuals and so are molecules. What is food for one is poison for another.

We are all unique individuals, it follows that no nutrition plan can be ideal for each one of us. Prepackaged diet plans are unsuitable for most people.

We all have unique patterns of molecular relatedness. We have different requirements for nutrients, food rotation and groupings.

Empiricism is the key word. We must find out about our food allergy and abnormal bowel responses. Next we must apply this knowledge and see for ourselves what works best for us. We learn what suits our molecules and tissues best by listening to our body tissues and by experimentation. I reiterate here what I wrote before:

Life span nutrition is about knowing our foods and their relationship to our lives.

The key word in the above statement is *knowing*. First, we must learn about foods. Next, we must understand the difference between foods that sustain us and so-called foods with which we stuff our bowels, but which do not preserve our health. It is only then that we will *know* the relationship between our food and our lives. I indicated earlier that appropriate tests for food allergy are very valuable. But the test results must be subordinated to our "intuitive" interpretation of these test results, very much like a physician interprets test results within the total context of a given case history.

SEVENTH, WE DIVERSIFY AND ROTATE OUR FOODS.

This is an essential issue not only for allergic individuals but for all people. I have sometimes wondered why nature created seasons and seasonal foods if it were not to ensure rotation and diversification of foods for living things. Of course, that was before we invented refrigerators and built glowing monuments to our love for hamburgers, french fries and milk shakes at every major intersection in the country.

I have never seen a child who was allergic to Brussels sprouts. I suppose the reason for this is that Brussels sprouts do not taste the way chocolate does. Allergy is a genetic predisposition. We are programmed to react to elements in our environment. That means there are two facets to this problem of allergy: genetic programming and exposure. The Swedish do not have ragweed allergy. When they come to the United States, they are usually sensitized the first year and develop symptoms of allergy in their second or third year in this country.

Rotary diversified nutrition was Nature's prescription for us. We need to return to that grand design. In the chapter Life Span Food Choices, I outlined in detail my recommendations for a rotary diversified diet.

EIGHTH, WE LEARN ABOUT NUTRIENT DENSITY

Nutrient density (quantity of nutrients in food) is drastically cut down by modern food processing. The major considerations in this context are:

Increased demand for food is disrupting the natural order in our food chain. Increased crop output is leaching the soil of its nutrient density. For a long time now, we Americans have prided

ourselves o being the bread basket of the
whole world. Little do we realize how we have
punished our soil to reach this goal.

. Increased shelf life of food is achieved by processing
which depletes the nutrient value of foods.

. Increased requirements of profitability of our fast food
outlets cause maladaptation of taste buds among
our children and adults.

. Increased appetite for any foods and all foods.

NINTH, WE LEARN AND PRACTICE Ph (ACID-ALKALI) BALANCE IN OUR FOOD

We all know something about how acid rain is ruining
the ecology of our forests. Rarely do we recognize that there is
a greater acid rain on our body tissues. I mentioned earlier in
this volume that spontaneity of oxidation is the basic equation
of life. Aging-oxidant molecules increase the oxidative stress and
cause premature aging. Life span molecules provide a
counterbalance and prevent premature aging. Oxidative
breakdown of foods in our body produces acid molecules. The
body tissues work hard to generate life span molecules to
neutralize this acidity.

Environmental chemical pollutants are powerful aging-
oxidant molecules. These are the molecules that the rain on our
forest acid. These are the molecules that leach toxic minerals
such as mercury and aluminum from the soil. These are the

molecules that "acid rain" on the molecules in our bodies.

Whenever possible we should know the following in making our food choices.

* Meats are acid ash foods.
* Grains are acid ash foods.
* Vegetables are alkaline ash foods.
* Fruits, with some exception, are alkaline ash foods.
* Our molecules are under a heavier acid rain than our forests.
* Our metabolism produces acidotic stress.
* Stress response increases acidotic stress.
* Environmental pollutants increase acidotic stress.
* A practical guide: Foods should be 80% alkaline ash and 20% acid ash types.
* Combine vegetables with grains or vegetables with meats, but not grains with meats. A side benefit of this strategy is improved digestion of food (meats require 3-4 hours for digestion, grains 1-2 hours and vegetables less than one hour).

The metabolic individuality of a person is a central issue in the way foods serve as life span or aging oxidative agents. Examples of this phenomenon include food allergy, food intolerance, deficiencies of digestive enzymes and nutritional deficiencies. Food allergy converts life span foods into aging-oxidant foods, and makes aging-oxidant foods more potent in their effects.

TENTH, WE EAT LIFE SPAN NUTRIENTS AND AVOID AGING-OXIDANT ELEMENTS

Life Span and Aging-Oxidant Sugars

In general, complex carbohydrates may be primarily regarded as life span sugars according to the criteria given in the preceding paragraphs. By contrast, simple carbohydrates may be primarily considered as aging-oxidant sugars.

Sugar is a major antinutrient in the American diet. Unfortunately, there is simply too much of this antinutrient in the American diet. I do not know how it came to pass that we Americans began to consider dessert an integral part of every meal. So-called low fat milk shakes generally contain as many as 320 calories, with as many as 250 calories in sugars. A piece of apple pie contains 260 calories, half in sugar and half in fats. Large quantities of sugar also enter our bodies in commercial cereals and as "hidden" sugar in such items as ketchup, salad dressings and most canned fruits.

Sugars exert their adverse effects in several ways, some of which I describe in the discussion of sudden hypoglycemia (low blood sugar) and hyperglycemia (high blood sugar) later in this chapter. Increased insulin activity caused by a high intake of sugars is a serious health hazard and has been implicated in the cause of heart disease, hypertension and strokes (see chapter On the Nature of Obesity). One other serious health hazard of excessive sugars in the diet concerns accelerated oxidative molecular injury. Simple sugars can produce free radicals by a chemical process called nonenzymatic glycosylation. Free radicals so produced add to the oxidative injury to proteins and fats in the body.

Whole wheat is an excellent source of complex carbohydrates. However, wheat allergy in my experience is a very common problem. Wheat substitutes are advisable for all people and are essential for people with wheat allergy. Brown rice, spelt, amaranth, quinoa, millet, komat, rye, oat and barley are excellent substitutes for wheat. Gluten sensitive people usually need to avoid rye, oat and barley.

Brown and wild rice take longer to cook but keep much better when cooked and frozen than most other foods. These are excellent sources of complex carbohydrates. Cook with some water left behind, add a small quantity of butter with raisins or fresh fruit. Reduce or eliminate milk with cereals.

Beans and lentils are other good sources of complex carbohydrates (as well as proteins). Beans provide lecithin to promote fat burning in the body and molybdenum for the life span enzymes included in the oxidase systems. Beans, greens, and grains support the life span bacterial flora in the gut that preserve life span enzymes.

Life Span and Aging-Oxidant Proteins

Natural unprocessed protein molecules can be considered as life span proteins, while processed, oxidized and denatured proteins can be considered aging-oxidant proteins. Meats, as is well known, are excellent sources of essential amino acids. However, we should recognize that meats also inhibit several life span enzymes such as the beta glucuronidase enzyme system. This causes the loss of such essential life span molecules as glutathione. Beans, nuts, lentils and whole grains are excellent sources of top-grade proteins. These foods are also excellent sources of minerals such as magnesium, potassium, calcium, zinc, iron, molybdenum and others. For instance, molybdenum serves as the life support mineral for oxidases and other enzyme systems.

Amino acid formulas (primarily protein products) composed of hydrolyzed amino acids and peptides with little or no sugar and fat content are excellent sources of amino acids, the building blocks for making proteins in the body. Amino acids are time-release energy foods. They prevent the molecular roller coasters caused by sugars. Good amino acid formulas can be taken with fresh vegetable juice, club soda, diluted soy milk or diluted rice milk. Unsalted canned vegetable juices and low-fructose fruit juices are other desirable alternatives.

Life Span and Aging-Oxidant Fats

The most common mistake we make in this area is that we focus on cutting down fats in our food but rarely pay attention to what kind of fats are present in our food. Good fats are essential for health. Cholesterol and its cousin, fat molecules *are* the guardian angels of our cell membranes, and the cell membrane is what separates internal order of the cell order from external disorder. Processed fats, hydrogenated oils and margarines are fats that contain substantial quantities of trans fatty acids, which we cannot metabolize, and other toxic cyclic by-products of processing methods.

A strategy of no oxidized fats is much more important than that of a low fat-diet. This must be regarded as the key issue in any consideration of fats in foods, health and disease.

"Nowhere in clinical medicine are the data so distorted to justify long-term drug therapy by practitioners of N^2D^2 medicine," Choua often says, "than in the area of cholesterol and its role in the cause of heart disease." Choua has his reasons for saying so.

I agree with Choua that cholesterol is by far the most maligned molecule in medicine today. It is mercilessly attacked by the proponents of the drug industry. It is misunderstood by the lay public. We physicians, in general, parrot the opinions of our cholesterol experts on the payroll of drug companies — not a bad example of echolalia in drug medicine. I discuss this subject at length in my monograph *Choua, Cholesterol Cats and Chelation.*

Low-fructose, low-acidity and high-fiber fruits

There are three important issues in eating fruits: 1) how much fructose (fruit sugar) they contain; 2) how much acid load fruits carry; and 3) the presence of fruit allergy. Oranges, grapes and bananas are among the fruits with high-fructose contents. The following three categories show relative acid load of common fruits.

   . Acid fruits: citrus fruits, pineapple, plums, strawberries, sour fruits, pomegranates.

   . Subacid fruits: apples, apricots, cherries, grapes, mangoes, papayas, pears.

   . Sweet fruits: bananas, dates, figs, prunes, raisins, persimmons.

Citrus fruits do have an overall alkaline effect. However, they can cause some initial additional acidotic burden. Recognition of fruit allergy requires allergy tests. In general, some fruits are more allergenic than others, for example allergy to orange is much more common than allergy to apples in my clinical practice. Sugar content of fruits is another important issue. Fructose is metabolized more slowly than glucose. Still it may add a considerable simple sugar overload and is poorly tolerated by many individuals with sugar sensitivity. A listing of first, second and third food choices is included in the chapter Life Span Food Choices.

We See the Snack Value in Nuts and Seeds

Nuts and seeds are excellent snacks. We should remember nature designed nuts and seeds to serve as the *whole* food for the plant before and during its birth. These foods are clearly the best sources of essential minerals such as calcium, magnesium, potassium, molybdenum, manganese, copper, selenium and iron.

It is essential to eat these snacks in rotation. Nuts are among the highly allergenic foods. I recommend that peanuts be avoided. A very large number of my patients with allergy are allergic to peanuts. We become allergic to foods that we eat most. Many of us were brought up on peanut butter and jelly sandwiches.

Nuts are also rich in fats. For example, peanut butter has 90% of its calories in fats. Thus, nuts as snacks should be eaten judiciously.

Desserts

* First choice: fruits eaten as desserts.
* Second choice: desserts prepared with fruit juices as sweeteners.
* Third choice: desserts prepared with Stevia extract and natural syrups.
* Fourth choice: desserts prepared with Aspartame (Nutrasweet) and saccharine (infrequent use for those without chemical sensitivity).

* Desserts should not be eaten regularly.
* Desserts should never be eaten as snacks or as a substitute for regular meal items. Doing so is the best way to throw ourselves into a metabolic roller coaster.
* Cakes, candy, cookies, creams, caramel and other common desserts should not be kept at home for company.

Life Span Fasting

Fasting is as old as man's history: There is cultural fasting. There is religious fasting. There is seasonal fasting. Finally, there is fasting as a medical remedy. There are different types of fasting, depending on the permissible materials (water fasting, vegetable juice fasting, fruit juice fasting and liquid fasting). There are also different types of fasting as regards the length of fasting (daytime fasting, all day fasting, week-long fasting, and extended fasting for months).

Sick animals refrain from eating. We consider this phenomenon instinctive. Throughout history, man reduced or stopped eating altogether when ill. This phenomenon is often regarded as intuitive. To me these phenomena are biologic adjustments that molecules, cells and tissues make without seeking prior clearance from our thinking minds. In medical jargon, we call them "pathophysiologic adaptations."

Sickness creates a host of self-perpetuating molecular roller coasters. In most cases, the initial factors that make us "not well" are minor and self-limiting. What converts these minor ailments (the dis-ease state) into major diseases are molecular roller coasters. A sick animal that refrains from eating and a sick person who stops eating do so for "molecular reasons." Molecules suppress hunger so food intake declines. As the factors that cause sickness subside, hunger returns to its normal level.

Fasting is an excellent way of understanding the impact of food allergy and chemical sensitivity upon health. This type of fasting usually requires pure water fasting for five or more days. Fasting for diagnostic purposes *must* be done under close knowledgeable professional supervision. Unsupervised fasting of this type can be dangerous, and I do not recommend it.

Life span fasting, by contrast, is done for long-term therapeutic benefits. The concept of fasting for the life span is based upon a basic premise: Fasting must be done in such a way as to foster good health for the expected life span. Following are some specific recommendations.

Cortical Fasting Vs Limbic Fasting

Cortical fasting is fasting with an overall analytical focus. It includes detailed plans for keeping busy throughout the day. It is a goal-oriented fasting, fasting to rid oneself of allergic foods, or to reduce chemical burden, or to think clearly.

When ye fast, be not, as the hypocrites, of a sad countenance.

Mathews 6:16

Limbic fasting is fasting with an inner visceral calm. It does not require a day plan. It is a day for just *being*. It is a day without goals and objectives. It is a time for rest, meditation and prayer. It is a time for the limbic state.

Limbic fast is a day without TV, and without household chores. It is a day without social events, without animated conversations, a day without household chores. Some of my patients have told me how difficult it is for them not to do anything even for brief periods of one half hour. That is one of the clearest signals of inner visceral turmoil. It calls for yet more time for just being there, more time for autoregulation. A life span fast must be a limbic fast.

What Do I Do During the Fast?

People often ask me this question. It is a revealing question. It shows that the person is worried about what he is going to do with himself during the period of fasting, solitude and silence.

Most of us seemingly yearn for some personal time. Indeed, this is the most frequent lament I hear. It is the principal price we pay for a life in "advanced" countries. Our technology has speeded up our lives. We recognize the full impact of it on our biology. And yet, the very prospect of some moments of solitude and silence raises the issue of what to do. We become uncomfortable with the thought of being by ourselves.

A day of life span fast should be a day of prayer, meditation autoregulation, and rest. Life span fast as described here should include ample time for rest and for frequent catnaps, which are extremely valuable for lowering the molecular thermostats and eliminating molecular roller coasters. Longer periods of sleep clearly indicate a need for additional sleep.

TV viewing should be scrupulously avoided. Soft music is fine but only for some of the time. Reading time should be kept short and reading should be of the light type. A life span fast should not be a day for heavy reading or reading materials that demand full attention.

Limbic Breathing

A day of life span fasting should be a day of limbic breathing. Two limbic breaths here, three limbic breaths there, all day long until it becomes a part of the day. Each limbic breath counts.

Duration of the Fast

One day at a time

Frequency of the Fast

One day a week or a fortnight

Type of Fast

Mixed vegetable and mixed fruit juice fasting

Colonics or Enema

None. Unless determined by the physician for some subacute medical contingency

C-Catharsis

"C-Catharsis" is a procedure for cleansing the bowel using progressively larger doses of vitamin C until a state of diarrhea is induced and the bowel movement is essentially composed of clear water. The quantities of vitamin C required may be as much as 20 to 60 grams. This is extremely valuable, but must be undertaken under close supervision of a professional.

C-catharsis is not essential for every fasting period. Ideally, it should be done on the day before the planned fasting. Uncommonly, loose bowel movements with C-catharsis may be associated with some cramps. If this does happen, it is a harmless temporary phenomenon.

Physical Activity During Fast

Not recommended for the first three times. Plan weekend days for extended rest and as little physical activity as possible, except for a 15-30 minute period of limbic exercise (walking or slow and sustained running with limbic breathing, without any muscle strain or fatigue).

Vegetable Juices

Vegetable juices should be prepared by using two or three vegetables at a time and drunk fresh. Here are some suggested combinations:

Carrots, celery and broccoli
Red beets, cucumber and spinach
Chinese cabbage, turnips and peas
String beans, parsley and asparagus

Give preference to First and Second Choice vegetables (see the chapter Life Span Food Choices. Carrot juice is excellent but not for daily consumption or for each time we fast. Similarly, tomato and peppers should be used sparingly. Vegetables with a pungent taste such as burdock, radish, garlic, mustard and onions should be added in small amounts according to personal taste.

The vegetable and fruit juices should be diluted with equal quantities of suitable water. Thus, each glass of vegetable or fruit juice should be drunk with an additional glass of water. Both glasses of diluted juices can be sipped slowly or all at once according to one's desire at that time.

Fruit Juices

Prepare fruit juices with First Choice Fruits (see the chapter Life Span Food Choices). Fruits in the Third Choice category should be avoided. These fruits are very acidic, very sweet and rich in fructose content, or have a high allergenic potential. Examples: orange, banana, grapes, mango.

Herbal Teas

Herbal teas make excellent drinks for fasting. All herbal teas included on page 275 may be taken in rotation. For my own patients, I compound a tea that includes fennel seed, fenugreek, licorice and Peau D'Arco. It has an excellent taste.

(Some of my patients initially did not like its taste the first time around. However, for most of them this was a temporary handicap.) These natural products have been used for centuries for their beneficial effects on the general state of metabolism and the internal conditions of the gut. One or two teaspoons of this protocol should be added to 4 cups of boiling water for five minutes. This tea can be taken hot or cold according to personal taste. It can be refrigerated and reheated without impunity. Other herbal teas are recommended in rotation. Herbal teas of medicinal value should not be taken except under professional supervision.

Guidelines for Fluids Intake During Fasting

8:00 am	2 cups of Herbal Protocol 1
	If desired, drink extra water with nutrients
	Meditation and autoregulation
9:00 am	1 glass of fresh vegetable juice
11:00 am	2 cups of Herbal Protocol 1
	Meditation and autoregulation
1:00 pm	1 glass of fresh life span fruit juice
2:00 pm	Rest, meditation and auto regulation
5:00 pm	1 glass of fresh life span fruit juice or one glass of broth
6:00 pm	2 cups of Herbal Protocol 1
	Walk limbically
	If desired, 1 glass of ginger root water

Meditation and autoregulation
Light reading in bed (poems,
spiritual writings or nature articles)

HYPOGLYCEMIA
and hyperglycemic, insulin and adrenergic surges

The clinical problems of hypoglycemia are complicated by the fact that lay people misunderstand the disorder, and patients may attempt to impose their views on the physicians.

Postgraduate Medicine July 1990

This is an illuminating statement. The first part of this statement concerns the nature of this problem. As a hospital pathologist, I have examined several thousand glucose tolerance test results. As a practicing nutritionist-physicians, I have cared for a very large number of patients who suffer from symptoms of weakness, jittery-ness, nausea, headache, sweating and heart palpitation that respond extremely well to nutritional management. It is my sense that hypoglycemia is misunderstood by physicians much more frequently than by the patients. Patients *know* something about this problem because they suffer from it. Physicians who do not practice nutritional medicine are incarcerated in a textbook model of thinking about this common metabolic problem which is simply irrelevant to the suffering caused by it.

The second part of this statement is equally interesting.

The author laments the fact that patients who suffer from this problem may attempt to impose their views on the physician. This fascinates me. In classical medicine, we physicians are brought up to be on guard against patients imposing their views on us. The unspoken principle here is that the physician knows everything, and the patient nothing. In my practice of molecular medicine, I *want* to be guided and influenced by my patient's views. After all, it is his tissues and body that I am working with. I can bring to the care of my patients the best in medical science and technology, but one thing I can never do is to get under his skin. Who is a better judge of what works and what does not, the patient or his physician? In matters of clinical observation in an acute illness, clearly the experienced physician is a better judge. When it comes to long-term management of chronic symptoms such as those caused by blood sugar roller coasters, my unequivocal answer is "patient." *This, to me, is one of the most fundamental difference between the classical drug medicine and the new molecular medicine.*

What is hypoglycemia?

Hypoglycemia, by definition, means low blood sugar.

Hypoglycemia is a widely misunderstood term. Some professionals regard it as a very uncommon clinical problem, while others consider it a common malady. The first group of professionals consider management of this problem in most cases as treatment of imaginary diseases (the old "all in the head story"). Professionals in the second group consider such opinions as based on ignorance.

According to medical texts, the diagnosis of hypoglycemia

should be made only when the blood sugar level of 50 mg/dl or lower is associated with symptoms of hypoglycemia (weakness, sudden mood swings, sweating, nausea, cramps, vomiting, light-headedness, heart palpitations and tremors). The frequency of hypoglycemia, as defined by the above classic criteria, is extremely low (less than one half percent in a series of 1500 glucose tolerance curves I have examined during the last several years). *Yet, the occurrence of symptoms associated with sudden shifts in blood sugar levels are quite common (about 20% in the above study).*

The hypoglycemia controversy is spurious. It arises from a failure to consider some elementary aspects of the glucose tolerance study. In our laboratory, we carefully explain to the patient the nature of the test and ask *the patient* to record the absence or presence of symptoms each time the blood sample is drawn and also if symptoms occur during the intervals between sampling. The significance of the glucose tolerance tests becomes quite apparent when this simple precaution is taken.

The symptoms that are usually considered "hypoglycemic" occur about nine times as frequently when the blood sugar level rises sharply than when it reaches its lowest point. This is the single most important insight I have gained from my rather extensive and careful personal study of this subject. This means that the so-called hypoglycemic symptoms actually occur much more frequently when the blood sugar level is actually rising. In other words, the symptoms of hypoglycemia (low blood sugar) are, in reality, the symptoms of hyperglycemia (high blood sugar). A similar relationship is observed between blood insulin levels and hypoglycemic symptoms. The absolute numerical value of the blood sugar level is of little significance (except when an insulin producing tumor drives the blood sugar value down to 20 or 30). The central issue in the hypoglycemia controversy is the *rate of change* in the blood sugar level. This is the crux of the matter.

How does a rapidly rising blood sugar level cause symptoms believed to be caused by hypoglycemia?

Sharp rises in the blood sugar level evoke sharp responses from the beta cells of the pancreas that release insulin. Sudden bursts of insulin cause a sudden release of adrenaline and its cousins, the adrenergic molecules. What we consider symptoms of hypoglycemia are, by and large, symptoms of hyperactive adrenergic responses (excess adrenaline). Some of these symptoms are also caused by the insulin overshoot phenomenon which drives the blood glucose level down to a level that cannot support the energy needs of the body.

A clear understanding of the relationship between the symptoms of hypoglycemia and the rate of change in the blood sugar level is essential for success in the management of hypoglycemia with a nutritional approach. *Prevention of hypoglycemic symptoms calls for a focus on the metabolic events that occur two to three hours before their development.* It requires a strategy for avoiding the glucose molecular roller coaster caused by heavy sudden overload of simple sugars. I cite an example to illustrate this sequence of events.

An eight-year-old child has a blood sugar level of 100 mg/dl (or 1,000 mg in one liter of blood). Since he has a total circulating blood volume of about 5 liters, the total quantity of glucose in his circulating blood is 5000 mg or 5 grams. A teaspoonful of sugar holds 4 grams of sugar. Now this boy drinks a can of soda that contains 8 to 10 teaspoonfuls of sugar. This means that by drinking a can of soda, that child pours six to eight times as much sugar into his blood as exists at any time. Such a massive overload of sugar throws him into a sugar roller coaster, followed by an insulin roller coaster, which in turn triggers an adrenaline roller coaster. Similar molecular roller coasters are caused when he drinks a 12-ounce glass of commercial orange juice. How is the sugar molecular roller coaster initiated? With sugar overload. How is the sugar molecular roller coaster perpetuated? By withdrawal symptoms. "Highs" in the blood sugar levels are followed by the "lows" that create biologic demands for yet more sugar. Sugar craving is another name for sugar addiction. An American child at the turn of the century consumed between 5 and 10 pounds of sugar per year. His counterpart today ingests 150-175 pounds. How many thousands of molecular roller coasters does that come to? The numbers add up. This is the essence of the hypoglycemia problem. How does our sugar industry respond to all this? They keep physicians on their payroll to publish absurd studies showing that our children are not hurt by sugar. This is the simple truth behind the hypoglycemia controversy.

Are there some other important factors in the cause of hypoglycemia?

Yes, there are the factors of food allergy that can cause, mimic or exaggerate molecular roller coasters caused by sugar overload. A factor of paramount importance is the lack of physical exercise that causes insulin resistance (tissues become less responsive to insulin). I discuss this subject at length in the companion volume, *The Ghoraa and Limbic Exercise*. Oxidized and denatured foods impair, paralyze or completely inhibit life span enzymes, and, quite literally, clog molecular wheels of our metabolism. A clogged metabolism increases the stress on the body's ability to cope with sugar overload. Finally, stress causes and increases the intensity of glucose roller coasters. Adrenaline is the principal stress hormone. I indicated earlier in this commentary that the symptoms of hypoglycemia are predominantly the symptoms of adrenaline.

How can the troublesome hypoglycemic-hyperglycemic shifts be prevented?

There are four basic strategies for the prevention of hypoglycemia: nutritional, allergy management, stress control and physical fitness. I discuss the subjects of food and mold allergy in my monograph, *In-Vitro Allergy: Diagnosis and Management.* I discuss methods for stress control, self-regulation, and physiological effects of limbic breathing in *The Cortical Monkey and Healing* and *The Limbic Dog and Directed Pulses.* The companion volume *The Ghoraa and Limbic Exercise* deals with exercise. I include below a brief outline of four nutritional strategies for preventing rapid hyperglycemic and hypoglycemic responses:

Four Strategies for Sugar Roller Coasters

People who suffer from sugar roller coasters should know that this metabolic disorder is entirely reversible. Initially, the person often needs to follow the management plan rigidly. As the metabolic enzyme functions are normalized, the molecular roller coasters subside and the normal molecular defenses gain strength. Rigidity in nutritional plans, in general, becomes unnecessary.

First,

Eat time-release energy foods. Avoid rapid fire energy foods.

High-protein and moderate fat foods are time-release energy foods. Foods can be supplemented with well-formulated peptide, amino acid and protein formulas. Some alkali supplements are very useful between meals to reduce the acidotic stress (my own alkali formulation includes the following: potassium bicarbonate, 40 mg; calcium carbonate, 35 mg; and magnesium carbonate, 120 mg. I recommend two tablets of this formulations mid-way between breakfast and lunch and two tablets mid-way between lunch and dinner).

Cakes, candy, cookies, colas, creams, caramel and sugary snacks are rapid fire foods. Even complex carbohydrates need to be avoided in severely symptomatic cases of hypoglycemic-hyperglycemic shifts.

Second,

Eat six small meals rather than three large ones.
Avoid starve-binge-starve cycles.
Never miss breakfast.
Stay over-hydrated at all times.

Third,

Aging-oxidant desserts must be avoided. Desserts prepared with fruit juices and sweeteners may be eaten infrequently and only after regular meals. The common practice of omitting the meal and "just eating the dessert" must be avoided at all costs. Desserts should be prepared as outlined earlier in this chapter. Table sugar must be avoided.

Fourth,

Avoid incompatible and allergic foods (as determined by electrodermal method, skin tests or other suitable blood IgE antibodies tests). Commonly used IgG test for the diagnosis of food allergy, in my judgment, is not the best choice.

FOOD CHOICES FOR HYPOGLYCEMIA

Our food choices for the prevention of rapid

hypoglycemic-hyperglycemic shifts should be made from a life span perspective. It is imperative that appropriate food allergy tests be performed and highly allergic foods be excluded. Optimal fluid intake is a critically important issue in the nutritional plan for this disorder.

Breakfast Choices

Protein, peptide and amino acid formulations (carbohydrates and fats should be less than 10% in calories)

Eggs and meats (excluding highly processed and fatty meats)

Steamed vegetables (1 tablespoon of miso in 3 cups of water)

Cheese and tofu products in moderation (if milk allergy does not exist)

Herbal teas (my favorite herbal tea formulation includes Pau D'Arco, fennel seeds, fenugreek and liquorice. Coffee, common black tea or decaffeinated coffee, in general, should be avoided).

Aspartame or saccharine should be avoided, but may be sparingly used if sweetener cannot be eliminated altogether on a short notice. With time, the use of sweeteners becomes unnecessary.

Whole-wheat toast, amaranth bread, bagel and oatmeal and other cereals without sugar may be included once or twice during the week. Breads and starches need to be excluded completely when the symptoms of hypoglycemia are severe.

Mid-Morning Choices

Time-release snacks (soy nuts, pumpkin seeds, sunflower seeds, sesame seeds, nuts in rotation, excluding peanuts).
Spring or mineral water, herbal tea.
Suitable protein and alkali formulations.

Lunch Choices

Steamed or stir-fried vegetables.
Choice One and Choice Two Meats.

Afternoon Choices

One portion of fruit from Choice One and Choice Two categories. Fruits need to avoided if severe symptoms of hypoglycemia persist.
Snacks included in the mid-morning choices.
Suitable protein, peptides, amino acids and alkali formulations may be repeated if symptoms persist.

Dinner Choices

Steamed or stir-fried vegetables (Choice One and Choice Two vegetables)
Meats as in lunch choices
Water, herbal tea or decaffeinated coffee (See comment in on breakfast choices).

Late Evening Choices

Same as midmorning choices. Protein and peptide products if symptoms develop during early morning hours.

PERSONAL CLINICAL PREFERENCES
FOR CHRONIC HEALTH DISORDERS

The principles and practice of life span nutrition described in this volume, in my view, are of utmost importance in the lives of people who suffer from persistent immune and degenerative disorders. In my clinical practice, I find that the philosophy of life span nutrition goes a long way in arresting disease processes and restoring health and optimal energy. However, such patients do require medical care by professionals well-informed in matters of nutrition, environment, stress and fitness. The patient himself needs to acquire a larger perspective of the energy dynamics in health and disease.

It is not my purpose in this volume to address the issues that practitioners of this new medicine — which I call molecular medicine — face in their clinical practices. I discuss those subjects in my other publications directed to professionals. To impart basic information to the general readers, however, I include below a list of my own clinical preferences in the management of people with chronic environmental, immune and degenerative disorders. These are intended as areas of focus for the reader's physician. If our objective is to go beyond the sheer symptom-suppressing therapies that form the prevailing mode of drug medicine in the United States, we need better understanding of the real issues involved. Below are the elements that are essential to management plans for individual persons for promoting better health and longer lives.

- Learning, understanding and *knowing* the basic molecular and energy dysfunctions that cause chronic immune and degenerative disorders, both for the physician and the patient.

- Holistic molecular relatedness in biology

- Molecular (metabolic) individuality of the person

- Oxidative stresses: external and internal

- Acidotic stresses and metabolic roller coasters

- Food incompatibilities and abnormal bowel responses

- Specific environmental triggers

- Altered states of bowel ecology

- Altered states of specific organ ecologies

- Life span nutrition in the kitchen

- Oligo-antigenic (hypoallergenic) and alkaline ash foods

- Nutrient support: oral and intravenous therapies

- Fun activities

- EDTA chelation for heavy metal overload

- Limbic exercise

- Autoregulation, meditation, prayer and language of silence

In the appendix, I include the addresses and telephone numbers of the American Academy of Environmental Medicine and the American College for Advancement in Medicine. The physician members of these two organizations, in general, practice medicine with clinical preferences that are very close to those listed above.

Life Span Nutrition Is a Study
of the Human Condition

I end this chapter with the same words with which I started it: *We are what we observe.*

Life span nutrition is not about martyrdom before we eat or guilt after it. Life span nutrition is a matter of limbic listening; it is neither denial of dieting nor euphoria of eating. Life span nutrition is about respecting our food so it can respect us.

Life span nutrition is not about "low-sugar," "no-sugar," "low-yeast," "no-yeast," "high-protein," "low-fat," "megavitamin," or "banana-grapefruit" diets. It is not about dieting. It is not about calorie counting. It is not about losing weight, though loss of excess weight occurs as a natural consequence of *knowing* the relationship between food and life.

What Is Food for One Is Poison for Another
When God Cast Me, He Threw Away the Mold

The ancients spoke the words in the first line. Someone intoxicated with the brew of the *New Age* cried out the words in the second line.

The ancients understood the metabolic uniqueness of

individuals. It is not simply a matter of allergy caused by IgE antibodies as is generally believed by the physician community. It is a matter of digestive enzymes and digestibility of foods, of absorptive capacity of the gut lining and the absorbability of broken down foods, of damaged gut ecology and overgrowth of disease-causing microbes, of constricted arteries and suffocated bowels, of detoxification enzymes and pollutant overload, and of life span enzymes and cellular health. Roger Williams, the well-known nutrition pioneer of our time, called it biochemical individuality. The basic chemistry of electrons and molecules is providing us new insights into matters of nutrition and health. Science is mapping out the territory intuitively seen by the ancients.

Nutrition courses, nutrition books, nutrition seminars and practicing nutritionist can only provide valuable guidelines. No one can truly determine the nutritional individuality of anyone else. This is one task that a person must do for herself or himself, *by learning, understanding, observing and knowing.*

There Is A Butterfly In Each One of Us — Each One of Us Has His Skylights

There are skylights of disbelief, skylights of misinformation and skylights of deception. Sometimes I see cracks in these skylights.

I see a crack in the skylight each time a child begins to recognize the relationship between what he eats and how he

feels. I see a crack in the skylight each time a young man feels
the brain fog lift as he avoids a chemical at work. I see a crack
in the skylight each time I see a woman with cold hands feel the
flash of warmth and energy that comes with successful self-
regulation. I see a crack in the skylight each time a woman
incapacitated by chronic fatigue regains her energy with nutrient
therapies. I see a crack in the skylight each time a man
challenges his physician who insists treatment of all diseases
must involve drugs or surgical scalpels. I see a crack in the
skylight each time someone defies the script prescribed by our
drug medicine. I see a crack in the skylight each time someone
refuses to accept a diagnostic label and begins his search for the
true causes of his affliction. I see a crack in the skylight each
time a holistic physician rises to defend his right to care for his
patients without drugs or surgery. I see a crack in the skylight
each time he fights back as his license is put in jeopardy by men
and women who sit on medical boards, under their own heavy
skylights of disbelief and obsolete notions of science in
medicine.

Everyday I see cracks in skylights.

Appendix

Physcian Associations
Dedicated to Preventive Medicine

Following is a listing for physician associations committed to preventive medicine. This is an excellent source for finding a physician in your area who is knowledgeable, experienced, and able to offer you good medical advice and help you reverse chronic nutritional, immune and degenerative disorders with non-drug therapies.

American Academy of Environmental Medicine
P.O.Box 16106
Denver, Colorado 80216
(303) 622-4224

American College of Advancement in Medicine
23121 Verdugo Drive, Suite 204
Laguna Hills, CA 92653
(714)583-7666

American Academy of Otolaryngic Allergy
Suite 303
1101 Vermont Ave, N.W.
Washington D.C. 2005

Foundation for Advancement in Medicine
P.O.Box 338
Kinderhook
New York 12106-0338
(800)-462-3246

Great Lakes Association of Clinical Medicine
70 W Huron Street
Chicago, Illinois 60610
(312) 266-7246

American Holistic Medical Association
4101 Lake Boon Trail, Suite 201
Raleigh, North Carolina 27607
(417) 865-5940

Recovery Inc.
802 No. Dearborn Street
Chicago, Illinois 60610
(312) 337-5661

Weight & Height Table for Men

HEIGHT	SMALL FRAME (+-3)	MEDIUM FRAME (+-5)	LARGE FRAME (+-6)
5'2"	128	132	140
5'3"	130	134	143
5'4"	132	136	145
5'5"	134	138	148
5'6"	136	141	151
5'7"	139	144	154
5'8"	141	147	158
5'9"	143	150	161
5'10"	146	153	165
5'11"	148	156	168
6"	150	159	172
6'1"	155	163	176
6'2"	158	167	180
6'3"	162	170	185
6'4"	166	175	190

RANGE	(+ - 7)	(+-8)	(+ - 12)

Weight & Height Table for Women

HEIGHT	SMALL FRAME (+-4)	MEDIUM FRAME (+-6)	LARGE FRAME (+-7)
4'10"	105	112	120
4'11"	106	114	123
5'	107	116	125
5'1"	110	119	128
5'2"	112	122	131
5'3"	115	125	135
5'4"	118	128	138
5'5"	121	131	142
5'6"	124	134	145
5'7"	127	137	149
5'8"	131	140	152
5'9"	133	143	155
5'10"	136	146	157
5'11"	139	149	161
6'	144	152	164
RANGE	(+-5)	(+-7)	(+-9)

Calories and Fat and salt Content of Foods
Generally Desirable Foods

Item	Portion	Cal	F	Na
Almonds, dried	12 med.	100	9	1
roasted and salted	12 med.	105	10	33
Applebutter	1 Tbs.	35	*	*
Apple juice	8 oz.	110	*	2
Apples:				
baked,				
w/2 Tbs. sugar	1 large	200	*	10
fresh, peeled	1 med.	70	*	1
Applesauce,				
sweetened	4 oz.	100	*	3
unsweetened	4 oz.	55	*	*
Apricot nectar	4 oz.	65	*	*
Apricots:				
can, light syrup	4 oz.	40	*	1
can, water pack	4 oz.	40	*	1
dried	3 small	60	*	6
fresh, whole	3	66	*	1
Artichoke, boiled,				
drained	1 avg.	50	*	45
Asparagus:				
boiled	6 spears	20	*	1
can, drained	6 spears	20	*	227
frozen	4 oz.	25	*	2
Avocado, raw	1/2 avg.	190	18	4
Banana	1 med.	95	*	1
Barley	4 oz.	390	1	5
Bass, baked &				
stuffed	4 oz.	280	18	100
Bass, fried	4 oz.	230	10	80

Bean sprouts, mung	4 oz.	40	*	5
Bean sprouts, soy	4 oz.	115	5	5
Beans, green:				
fresh, cooked	1 cup	30	*	8
frozen or raw	4 oz.	40	*	8
Beans, kidney				
cooked	1 cup	225	*	6
Beans, lima:				
dried	4 oz.	391	1	4
fresh	4 oz.	135	*	2
Beans, pinto, raw	1/2 cup	390	1	1-
cooked, no salt	1 cup	266	1	15
Beef, cooked:				
broiled, lean	4 oz.	254	12	68
broiled, lean				
and fat	4 oz.	528	48	68
flank, braised	4 oz.	223	8	68
ground beef				
(hamburger), lean	4 oz.	248	13	55
ground beef				
(hamburger), reg.	4 oz.	325	23	53
Beet greens	1 cup	25	*	105
Beets, raw	4 oz.	50	*	70
Beverages:				
Beer	12 oz.	151	0	25
Lite beer	12 oz.	96	0	*
Distilled Liquors				
(Gin, Rum, Vodka,				
Whiskey)				
80 proof	2 fl. oz.	130	0	1
86 proof	2 fl. oz.	140	0	1
90 proof	2 fl. oz.	154	0	1
Wine:				
Table (12.2 alcohol)	4 oz.	100	0	5
Milk:				
Skimmed	1 cup	85	*	123
Orange juice	1 cup	110	*	2
Soft drinks, diet	12 oz.	1	0	60

Soft drinks, regular	12 oz.	157	0	*
Water	1 cup	0	0	2
Blackberries	1 cup	60	*	1
Blackberry juice	1 cup	80	*	2
Black-eyed peas	4 oz.	83	*	33
Blueberries, fresh	1 cup	60	*	1
Bran, wheat	1 oz.	60	1	3
Bread:				
French	1 slice	50	*	100
Italian	1 slice	60	*	127
pumpernickel	1 slice	70	*	182
raisin	1 slice	65	*	91
rye	1 slice	75	*	172
white	1 slice	65	*	122
whole wheat	1 slice	65	*	14
Breadcrumbs,				
dry, grated	1 Tbs.	25	*	47
Broccoli, fresh	4 oz.	30	*	15
Broccoli, frozen	4 oz.	35	*	15
Brussel sprouts,				
cooked	1 cup	50	*	15
Butter, unsalted	1 Tbs.	100	11	2
Buttermilk	1 cup	85	*	307
Cabbage, boiled	1/2 cup	16	*	12
Cabbage, Chinese	4 oz.	15	*	24
Cabbage, coleslaw	4 oz.	110	9	125
Cabbage, raw, shredded	1 cup	25	*	20
Cakes:				
angel food	1/12	135	*	142
fruitcake, dark,				
2" x 2" x 1/2"	1	114	4	47
Cantaloupe	1/4 melon	35	*	14
Carrots, raw	1 cup	45	*	50
frozen	1 cup	50	*	28
Cashew nuts, unsalted	2 oz.	335	26	9
Catsup, low sodium	1 Tbs.	15	*	4
Cauliflower, raw				
or boiled	1 cup	30	*	14

Celery, raw	1 cup	20	*	151
cooked	1 cup	21	*	132
Cereal:				
Puffed rice	1 cup	55	*	1
Puffed wheat	1 cup	54	*	1
Cheese:				
Cottage, creamed	1 oz.	30	1	65
with skim milk	1 oz.	25	*	84
Cherries:				
sweet in light syrup	1 cup	90	*	1
sour in light syrup	1 cup	100	*	1
fresh	1 cup	85	*	2
Chestnuts, dried	8 med.	50	1	1
Chestnuts, fresh	4 oz.	220	2	7
Chicken:				
fryer - baked:				
dark meat w/skin	4 oz.	189	7	98
dark meat	4 oz.	160	4	98
light meat w/skin	4 oz.	266	11	75
light meat	4 oz.	224	7	68
Chickpeas, dry	4 oz.	390	5	28
Chives	1 oz.	5	*	*
Clams:				
broiled	6	115	6	181
canned, drained	4 oz.	105	3	166
cherrystone	6	100	2	157
raw	4 oz.	135	6	142
steamed	4 oz.	100	3	157
Coconut:				
fresh	2 oz.	210	20	14
unsweetened	1/2 cup	305	30	25
Coffee, black	1 cup	30	3	8
Collards	1/2 cup	45	2	43
Cookies:				
Arrowroot	1	25	1	12
Coconut macaroons	2 small	100	5	42
Oatmeal	1 large	90	3	76

Peanut	1	65	2	24
Scotch shortbread	1	35	2	4
Sugar	1 med.	50	2	36
Vanilla wafer	1	25	1	14
Corn:				
boiled, fresh on the				
cob	1 small	75	1	*
Cornmeal	1/2 cup	230	2	1
Cornstarch	1 Tbs.	30	1	
Crab meat:				
frozen	1/2 cup	70	2	1
Crabapples	1 large	90	*	1
Crackers:				
Zwieback	5 pieces	155	4	30
Cranberries	4 oz.	52	*	2
Cranberry juice	4 oz.	75	*	1
Cranberry sauce	1 Tbs.	50	*	*
Cranberry relish	1 Tbs.	65	*	*
Cream:				
sour	2 Tbs.	61	5	10
Creamer, non-dairy	1 tsp.	11	1	11
Cucumber	8 inch	15	0	6
Dandelion greens				
cooked	4 oz.	40	*	53
Dates, dried, pitted	1/2 cup	280	*	1
Duck, roasted	4 oz.	190	9	75
Eggs:				
boiled or poached	1	80	6	133
fried	1	95	8	149
Egg yolk	1	10	0	29
Eggplant, boiled	1 cup	38	*	6
Endive or escarole	8 oz.	50	*	35
Figs:				
canned	4 oz.	75	*	4
dried	4	232	*	7
fresh	4 small	100	*	2
Flounder, raw	4 oz.	90	*	106

Flour:				
all purpose	1 cup	400	1	2
corn meal	1 cup	460	4	2
rye, dark	1 cup	410	3	1
rye, light	1 cup	440	1	1
soy bean, defatted	1 cup	313	6	1
whole wheat	1 cup	350	2	3
Fruit cocktail, canned	1 cup	190	*	26
fresh	1 cup	75	*	3
Fruit punch	1 cup	180	*	7
Garlic clove	1	5	*	1
Gelatin:				
Knox, powder	1 envelope	28	0	0
Jell-O	1/2 cup	81	*	46
Gooseberries	1 cup	60	*	2
Grape juice	1 cup	150	*	2
Grapefruit, fresh	1/2	75	*	10
Grapefruit juice	1 cup	90	*	2
Gum, chewing, regular	1 stick	8	0	*
Haddock, broiled	4 oz.	135	6	101
smoked	4 oz.	120	1	90
Halibut	4 oz.	200	9	157
Ham:				
broiled	1 oz.	75	6	13
Honey	1 Tbs.	65	0	1
Honeydew melon	2" wedge	50	0	18
Ice cream	1 scoop	150	9	29
Ice milk	1/2 cup	180	6	89
Ices	1 scoop	120	*	*
Jams & preserves	1 Tbs.	55	*	3
Jellies	1 Tbs.	55	*	5
Kale	4 oz.	51	*	72
Kohlrabi, boiled	4 oz.	27	*	8
Lamb, roasted leg of	4 oz.	320	20	79
Leeks	1 piece	7	*	1
Lemon, 2" diameter	1	20	*	1
Lemon juice	1 Tbs.	5	*	*

Lentils, baked	1 cup	210	*	19
Lettuce	2 leaves	7	*	5
Lichee nuts, dried	1 oz.	65	*	1
Lime, 1/2" diameter	1	20	*	1
Lime juice, fresh	1 cup	60	*	2
Liver, chicken	4 oz.	185	5	69
Loganberries, fresh	1 cup	90	*	1
canned	1 cup	160	*	4
Macaroni, cooked	4 oz.	125	*	1
Mangos	4 oz.	75	*	8
Marmalade	1 Tbs.	55	*	3
Melon balls	1 cup	55	*	3
Milk:				
dried, skimmed	1 Tbs.	30	*	44
dried, whole	1 Tbs.	40	2	32
goat's	1/2 cup	90	5	46
skimmed, no fat	1 cup	85	*	123
1% fat	1 cup	100	2	130
Molasses	1/4 cup	207	*	12
Mushrooms, raw	4 oz.	35	*	19
Nectarines	1	40	*	4
Noodles, egg, cooked	1 cup	200	2	3
Okra, raw	1 cup	50	*	4
cooked	1 cup	46	*	4
Onion, raw	1 avg.	40	*	11
cooked	1 cup	60	*	14
Onion, green	6	20	*	2
Orange juice:				
canned or frozen	1 cup	120	*	3
fresh	1 cup	110	1	2
Papaya, raw	1 cup	70	*	1
Parsley, fresh	1 Tbs.	1	*	1
Parsnips, cooked	1 cup	100	1	12
Passion fruit	4 oz.	102	*	32
Peaches:				
canned in heavy syrup	1 cup	200	*	5
canned in water	1 cup	75	*	5
dried, uncooked	1 cup	420	1	26

raw, sliced	1 cup	65	*	2
Pears, raw 3" long	1	100	*	3
Pears, canned	1 cup	195	1	3
Pear juice nectar	1 cup	195	1	3
Peas, fresh, cooked	1/2 cup	55	*	10
Peas, dried, cooked	4 oz.	85	*	10
Peppers, green fresh	1 med.	13	*	12
Persimmons	1 avg.	100	*	8
Pineapple:				
canned in heavy syrup	1 slice	50	*	1
fresh	1 cup	75	*	2
Pineapple juice	1 cup	135	*	2
Plums, fresh 2"	1	25	*	1
canned	1 cup	205	*	9
Pomegranate, raw	1 pound	160		8
Popcorn, popped, plain	1 cup	55	1	*
Pork:				
chops, baked/broiled	1 med.	275	16	50
roast, lean	3 oz.	196	11	55
Potatoes, white:				
baked	1 med.	90	*	4
boiled	1 med.	80	*	3
Prune juice	4 oz.	95	*	2
Prunes:				
dried	4	100	*	3
stewed without sugar	4 oz.	165	*	6
Pudding, rice	1/2 cup	165	3	94
vanilla	1/2 cup	143	5	84
Pumpkin, canned	1 cup	80	1	5
Radishes	4 small	8	*	8
Raisins	1/2 cup	240	*	22
Raspberries, fresh	1 cup	80	2	1
Red snapper, raw	4 oz.	100	1	72
Rhubarb, raw	1 cup	18	*	2
cooked w/sugar	1 cup	385	*	5
Rice,				
instant white cooked	1/2 cup	90	*	1
raw white	1/2 cup	335	*	5

Rutabaga, boiled	1/2 cup	40	*	5
Salad dressing:			
French	1 Tbs.	66	6	105
Thousand Island	1 Tbs.	70	7	112
Salmon, raw	4 oz.	250	19	51
Scallions	5	20	*	1
Sesame seeds	1 oz.	165	14	18
Shad, baked	4 oz.	225	13	88
Sherbets	1 scoop	130	1	10
Shortening	1 Tbs.	126	14	0
Shrimp cocktail	6 med.	75	1	2
Sole, fillet broiled	4 oz.	90	*	88
Spaghetti, cooked	1 cup	155	1	1
Spinach, cooked fresh	1 cup	40	1	86
Squash, cooked summer	1 cup	30	*	2
cooked, winter	1 cup	130	1	2
Strawberries, raw	1 cup	55	1	1
Sugar, granulated	1/2 cup	355	0	1
brown	1/2 cup	206	0	33
Sweet potatoes:			
baked	1 med.	155	1	13
boiled	1 med.	170	1	15
Syrups:			
caramel	1 Tbs.	65	0	*
corn	1 Tbs.	50	*	14
maple	1 Tbs.	50	0	2
molasses, medium	1 Tbs.	50	*	7
sorghum	1 Tbs.	55	*	13
Tangerine	1 med.	40	*	2
Tangerine juice	1 cup	125	1	3
Tea	1 cup	2	*	*
Tomato paste, canned	6 oz.	140	*	65
Tomatoes, fresh	1 med.	40	*	5
Turkey, all white meat	4 oz.	200	4	93
Venison, raw, lean	4 oz.	143	7	60

Vinegar	2 Tbs.	5	*	*
Water, tap	1 cup	0	0	2
Watermelon, 3/4"x10"	1 slice	84	1	4
Wheat bran	1 Tbs.	19	*	1
regular flakes	1 Tbs.	14	*	1
Yeast, bakers, dry	1 oz.	85	*	16
Yeast, brewers, dry	1 Tbs.	50	*	21
Yogurt, skimmed milk	1 cup	125	4	128
made w/whole milk	1 cup	150	8	114
skim milk & fruit	*1 cup*	*250*	*4*	*130*

Calories and Fat and salt Content of Foods
Generally Undesirable Foods

Item	Portion	Cal	F	Na
Anchovy paste	2 Tbs.	100	6	3,080
Apple brown betty	4 oz.	171	4	174
Bacon, Canadian	2 oz.	155	10	1,430
Bacon, crisp	3 strips	100	8	163
Bacon fat	1 tsp.	100	5	40
Baking powder	1 tsp.	6	*	386
Barbecue sauce	1 Tbs.	50	5	200
Beans, baked				
w/pork & molasses	4 oz.	170	5	430
w/pork & tomato	4 oz.	140	3	525
Beans, green: canned	1 cup	30	*	536
Beans, lima:				
canned, drained	4 oz.	80	*	205
Beans, wax, canned	4 oz.	30	*	146
Beef, corned	4 oz.	423	35	1,973
fillet mignon	4 oz.	516	46	68
Beef Pot Pie, baked	4" dia.	527	31	607

Beets, canned	4 oz.	35	*	236
Cocktails:				
w/club soda or tomato				
juice	5 fl. oz.	200	*	200
Pina Colada	2 fl. oz.	240	*	2
Cooking sherry	4 oz.	38	o	600
Dessert (18.8%				
alcohol)	4 oz.	100	0	5
Milk:				
whole	1 cup	170	10	131
Soft drinks, reg.	12 oz.	157	0	*
V-8 Vegetable juice	1 cup	45	*	872
Big Mac Hamburger	1	541	31	962
Biscuit, baking powder	1 2" dia.	103	5	171
Bologna	2 oz.	165	14	705
Bouillon cube	1	5	*	400
Brazilnuts	2 oz.	365	35	1
Bread sweet:				
banana nut	1 slice	185	2	212
date nut	1 slice	100	1	155
Bread sticks	1 oz.	86	*	444
Bread stuffing mix	1/2 cup	118	1	647
Bulger, canned	1 cup	246	5	621
Butter, salted	1 Tbs.	100	11	2
Cakes:				
applesauce	3 oz.	400	12	368
cheese cake, graham				
cracker crust	1/8 cake	510	25	347
chocolate, iced	4 oz.	345	9	220
cupcake, iced (1.8oz)	1	184	6	168
upside-down	1/9	275	10	360
Candy:				
almond chocolate bar	1 oz.	150	10	22
butterscotch	1 oz.	120	3	94
caramel	1 med.	60	3	34
chocolate, bitter or				
baking	1 oz.	145	15	1

milk, semi-sweet	1 oz.	145	9	26
fudge	1 oz.	120	4	57
hard candy	1 oz.	110	*	9
jelly beans	1 oz.	104	0	3
marshmallows	1 ave.	25	0	3
peanut brittle,				
no salt	1 oz.	120	3	9
raisins, chocolate				
covered	1 oz.	120	4	18
Candy bars				
Almond Joy	1 oz.	132	7	40
Baby Ruth	1 oz.	135	5	100
Butterfingers	1 oz.	134	5	93
Caravelle	1 oz.	127	5	50
Kisses, Hershey	1 piece	25	1	5
Licorice, black	1 oz.	100	2	30
Life Savers	5 pieces	45	*	5
Mars Bar	1 oz.	130	7	56
Mint Pattie	1 piece	50	1	3
M & M's	1 oz.	140	7	56
Peanut Butter Cup	1 oz.	143	7	99
Snickers	1 oz.	130	8	100
3 Musketeers	1 oz.	120	4	20
Toffee	1 piece	28	1	90
Carnation Instant				
Breakfast w/skim milk	1 cup	387	3	415
Carrots, canned	1 cup	45	*	354
Cashew nuts, salted	2 oz.	335	26	119
Catsup, regular pack	1 Tbs.	15	*	147
Cereal:				
Buckwheat	1 cup	102	1	264
Cheerios	1 cup	112	*	256
Corn Chex	1/4 cup	111	*	304
Corn flakes	1 cup	95	*	201
Granola, Nature				
Valley	1/3 cup	150	6	218
Grape Nuts	1/4 cup	104	*	147
Raisin Bran	1/2 cup	102	*	190

Rice Chex	1 cup	98	*	228
Cheese:				
Monterey Jack	1 oz.	102	8	204
Mozzarella	1 oz.	84	7	227
Parmesan, dry grated	1 oz.	105	7	247
Roquefort	1 oz.	105	8	465
Cheese fondue	4 oz.	315	21	615
Cheese omelet	2 eggs	260	21	434
Cheese souffle	1/2 cup	240	19	400
Cheese spreads	1 oz.	82	6	461
Cheeries, maraschino	2	10	*	
Chicken:				
barbecued or broiled	4 oz.	225	14	310
fryer - fried				
dark meat w/skin	4 oz.	299	15	90
dark meat	4 oz.	249	11	88
light meat w/skin	4 oz.	266	11	75
light meat	4 oz.	224	7	68
Chicken pie	4 oz.	225	13	245
Chip beef	2 oz.	110	4	2,330
Chili with beans	1 cup	335	15	1,337
Chili without beans	1 cup	510	38	1,693
Chili powder	1 tsp.	17	0	79
Chop Suey:				
chicken or pork	1 cup	120	6	1,067
vegetable	1 cup	112	6	995
Chow Mein:				
chicken or pork	4 oz.	115	4	323
Citron, candied	2 oz.	180	*	166
Clams:				
fried	6	200	15	525
roasted	6	135	6	213
Clam chowder	1 cup	102	4	1,055
Cocktail sauce	1 oz.	31	*	340
Cocoa, w/skim milk	1 cup	130	*	190
Cocoa, w/whole milk	1 cup	165	7	161
Cocoa syrup	1 Tbs.	40	*	110
Coconut:				

sweetened	1/2 cup	252	18	136
Coffee w/cream & sugar	1 cup	50	3	8
Cookies:				
Animal crackers	6	50	1	72
Brownies	1 oz.	119	8	
Butterscotch	1	140	8	161
Chocolate chip	3 med.	150	6	115
Fig Newtons	2	100	1	193
Ginger snaps	5	165	10	224
Graham Crackers	3 med.	75	2	141
Corn:				
cream style	1/2 cup	95	1	273
niblets	1/2 cup	95	1	318
Corn chips	1 oz.	164	11	160
Corn grits, cooked	1/2 cup	55	*	221
Cornbread	2 oz.	170	5	516
Crab meat, canned	3 oz.	85	2	842
Cracker meal	2 oz.	265	6	664
Crackers:				
Saltine	5 squares	61	2	156
Soda	5 squares	120	4	300
Cream:				
Half & Half	1/2 cup	160	13	55
Heavy	1 Tbs.	50	5	5
Light	1/2 cup	235	23	28
Croutons	12 avg.	70	4	176
Croissant rolls	1 tiny	254	10	
Danish pastry	2 oz.	240	13	208
Doughnut, plain	1 oz.	120	7	102
Eggs:				
deviled	2	225	15	244
scrambled	2	160	12	230
Egg white	1	10	0	29
Flour:				
Bisquick	1 cup	503	17	1,476
self rising, sifted and spooned	1 cup	373	1	1,144
Goose, roasted	4 oz.	480	41	255

Gravy	2 Tbs.	50	4	93
Haddock:				
fried, breaded	4 oz.	180	7	193
Ham:				
baked	4 oz.	320	25	55
canned, boneless	4 oz.	215	14	13
Ice cream sundae	1 avg.	450	25	97
Knockwurst	2 oz.	155	13	550
Lamb chop, broiled	4 oz.	476	42	79
Liver:				
beef, fried	4 oz.	260	12	209
calves, fried	4 oz.	290	15	134
Liver paste	2 oz.	260	25	420
Liverwurst	2 oz.	170	15	550
Lobster, baked/broiled	4 oz.	125	*	275
MSG (mono sodium glutamate)	1 tsp.	0	0	742
Macadamia nuts	2 oz.	390	40	0
Macaroni & cheese	1 cup	465	24	1,086
Macaroni salad	1 cup	26	20	150
Mackerel, broiled	4 oz.	265	17	120
canned	4 oz.	190	12	240
Margarine, regular	1 Tbs.	100	11	137
Mayonnaise	1 Tbs.	90	10	127
Meat loaf	4 oz.	225	15	127
Milk:				
buttermilk	1 cup	85	*	307
Evaporated	1/2 cup	113	4	97
malted	1 cup	235	10	206
whole milk	1 cup	170	10	131
Muffins, 3" diameter	1	120	4	180
Mushrooms, broiled				
with butter	4 oz.	65	5	923
canned	1 cup	40	*	941
Mustard	1 Tbs.	10	*	167
Oils, all	1/4 cup	487	54	0
Olives, green	4 med.	15	2	310
Omelet	2 egg	150	12	223

Onion rings	2 oz.	168	15	415
Oysters, canned	4 oz.	86	1	250
fried	4 oz.	270	16	233
raw	1 cup	160	4	177
Pancake, 4 "	1	60	2	110
Peanut butter	1 Tbs.	95	8	98
Peanuts, roasted				
and salted	1/2 cup	760	65	780
Peas, green, canned	1/2 cup	75	*	268
Pecans, halves	1 cup	740	70	*
Pickles:				
cucumber	4 spears	25	*	230
dill or sour	1 large	10	*	1,298
sweet	1 small	20	*	119
Pickle relish	1 Tbs.	12	*	62
Pies:				
apple or cherry	4" wedge	350	15	411
lemon meringue	4" wedge	305	12	337
pumpkin	4" wedge	275	15	279
strawberry	4" wedge	340	9	333
Pig's feet, pickled	4 oz.	225	16	1,000
Pine nuts	2 oz.	310	27	180
Pistachio nuts	16	50	5	32
Pizza, cheese	6" wedge	185	6	550
Popcorn w/butter, salt	1 cup	155	12	659
Potato chips	10 chips	115	8	200
Potatoes, french fry	10 pieces	155	7	133
mashed w/milk	1 cup	125	1	579
Pretzels, thin twisted	2	46	1	202
Pudding:				
bread	1/2 cup	210	7	279
tapioca	1/2 cup	110	4	128
Rice, brown	1/2 cup	78	*	357
Rice, white	1/2 cup	112	1	357
Salad dressing:				
bleu cheese	1 Tbs.	75	7	164
Italian	1 Tbs.	83	8	314
Roquefort	1 Tbs.	76	8	164

Russian	1 Tbs.	74	8	130
Salami	1 oz.	120	11	425
Salmon, canned	4 oz.	250	15	505
Sardines, canned	4 oz.	230	12	932
Sauerkraut	1/2 cup	25	*	1,037
Sausage, canned pork	4 oz.	425	37	1,784
Scallops, broiled	4 oz.	140	2	231
Shrimp, broiled	4 oz.	90	1	139
canned	3 oz.	100	1	321
Soup:				
bean	1 cup	170	6	1,023
beef broth	1 cup	30	1	325
chicken noodle	1 cup	55	2	863
clam chowder	1 cup	95	6	766
lentil	1 cup	180	2	566
minestrone	1 cup	105	3	991
split pea	1 cup	145	3	1,004
vegetable	1 cup	80	2	885
Soy beans, cooked	1 cup	234	10	536
Spaghetti, cooked with meat ball and tomato sauce	1 cup	330	12	1,002
Spaghetti sauce	1 cup	220	8	1,508
Spinach, canned	1 cup	45	1	443
Stew,, chicken	1 cup	166	6	1,018
Sweet potatoes canned	1 cup	235	*	99
Swordfish, broiled	4 oz.	200	8	140
Tomato juice	1 cup	45	*	474
Tomato puree, canned	4 oz.	50	*	
Tomatoes, canned or stewed	1 cup	50	1	310
Tortilla, corn	1	55	1	158
flour	1	214	7	192
Tuna, canned in oil	3 1/4 oz.	184	8	511
canned in water	3 1/4 oz.	112	2	553
Turkey, roasted	4 oz.	250	11	171
all dark meat	4 oz.	230	9	121
V-8 juice	1 cup	45	*	872

Veal chop	1 med.	260	15	97
Veal roast	4 oz.	245	19	91
Waffles, plain	1 med.	225	12	561
Water, artificially softened	1 cup	0	0	147
Whitefish, baked	4 oz.	210	16	246
Wienerschnitzel	7 oz.	480	21	240

Caloric Requirements For Men

WEIGHT	HEAVY	MEDIUM	LOW
110	2,200	2,000	1,850
121	2,350	2,000	1,850
132	2,500	2,300	2,100
143	2,650	2,400	2,200
154	2,800	2,600	2,400
165	2,900	2,700	2,500
176	3,050	2,800	2,600
187	3,200	2,950	2,700
198	3,350	3,100	2,800
209	3,500	3,200	2,900
220	3,700	3,400	3,100

Caloric Requirements For Women

WEIGHT	HEAVY	MEDIUM	LOW
88	1,550	1,450	1,300
99	1,700	1,550	1,450
110	1,800	1,650	1,500
121	1,950	1,800	1,650
128	2,000	1,850	1,700
132	2,050	1,900	1,700
143	2,200	2,000	1,850
154	2,300	2,100	1,950

Recommended Dietary Allowances
Seventh Edition, 1968, National Academy of Sciences

Index

ORDER FORM

Other books, monographs and tapes by Majid Ali

BOOKS

The Cortical Monkey and Healing
The Ghoraa and Limbic Exercise
The Canary and Chronic Fatigue
The Limbic Dog and Directed Pulses

MONOGRAPHS

Intravenous Nutrient Protocols for
Molecular Medicine
The Altered States of Bowel Ecology and
Health Preservation
Choua, Cholesterol Cats and Chelation

TAPES

Autoregulation (set of 2 tapes)
Life Span Nutrition (set of 4 tapes)
Chronic Fatigue: Diagnosis and
Management

LIFE SPAN HEALTH LETTER

To order, write to

IPM PRESS
95 East Main Street
Denville, New Jersey 07834
Or call (201) 586-4111

In praise of Ali's *The Cortical Monkey and Healing*

" .... people who read this book will benefit from it." Linus Pauling

"If anyone else told me of Majid Ali's dictum, I would disbelieve it all. Majid's expertise in so many fields makes disregarding anything he says a costly mistake. He has taught me autoregulation, and I have personally seen what it alone can do."

Hueston King, M.D., Past President
American Academy of Otolaryngic Allergy

"This is a fascinating book coming from a physician who was a surgeon who became a pathologist, immunologist, allergist, ecologist, and now a teacher in self-regulation. There are many little gems here."

Norman Shealy, M.D., Past President
American Holistic Medical Association

"The new book ... is a wonderful overview of the problems with "standard medical care." Dr. Ali mixes fact with philosophy into a unique and readable book. One can now clearly understand the illogic of "modern medicine" and the logic of "molecular medicine."

James Frackleton, M.D., Past President
American College for Advancement in Medicine

"It contains many fresh insights and much common sense. I intend to use it as a primary reference during my medical students teaching sessions this fall."

Jessica Davis, M.D.
Cornell Medical Center, New York